8-WEEK BLOOD SUGAR DIET COOKBOOK

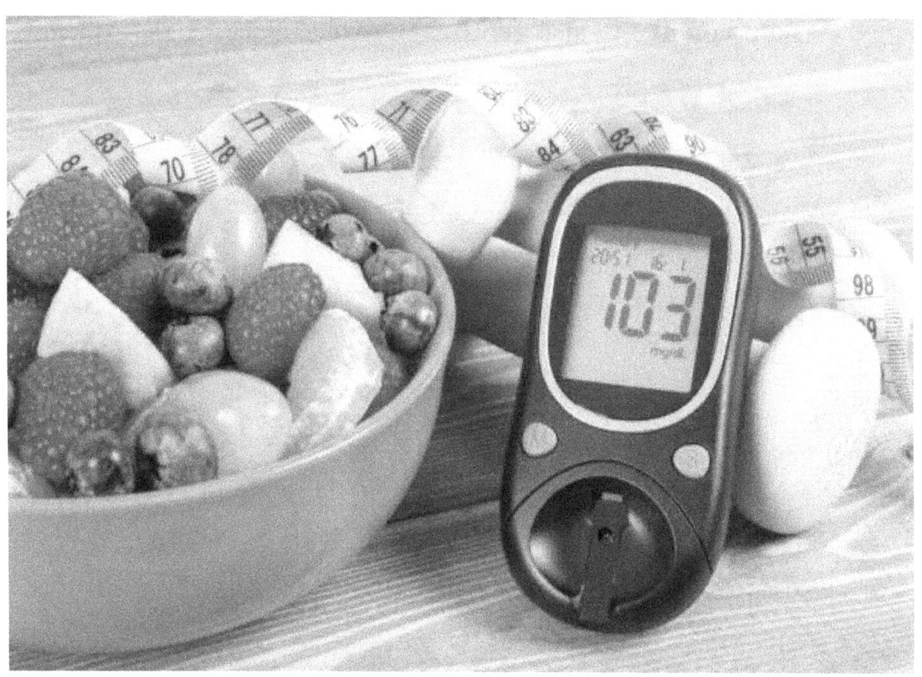

Dr. Samuel Jackson

Copyright (c) 2023 Dr. Samuel Jackson

Would you like to also get the following books by the Author

MEDITERRANEAN DIET COOKBOOK FOR BEGINNERS

CANCER DIET COOKBOOK FOR NEWLY DIAGNOSED

BREAST CANCER DIET COOKBOOK FOR NEWLY DIAGNOSED

BREAST CANCER DIET COOKBOOK FOR BEGINNERS

TABLE OF CONTENTS

INTRODUCTION

Before you go on to read this book, I want to tell you about Sarah.

Sarah had been struggling with diabetes for several years. She had tried all sorts of treatments, from insulin injections to oral medications, but nothing seemed to work for her. Her condition only seemed to be getting worse, and she was starting to lose hope.

One day, while browsing through Amazon kindle, Sarah came across my blood sugar diet cookbook (this very one you are reading now). Before this time, she had heard about the benefits of changing her diet to help manage her diabetes, so she decided to give it a try. She started following the recipes in my cookbook, carefully tracking her blood sugar levels every step of the way.

At first, Sarah found it difficult to stick to the (new) diet provided in this book. She had to give up many of her favorite foods and learn to cook with new ingredients that she had never used before. However, as she started to see improvements in her blood sugar levels, she became more motivated to keep going.

Over time, Sarah's diabetes began to improve dramatically. Her blood sugar levels became more stable, and she was able to reduce her reliance on medication. She even started to feel better overall, with more energy and fewer mood swings.

Eventually, Sarah's diabetes was completely cured, thanks to this blood sugar diet cookbook. She was overjoyed to be free of the burden of her illness and grateful to have found a solution that worked for her. She continued to follow the recipes in the cookbook and even started to experiment with her own healthy recipes, sharing her success with others who were struggling with diabetes.

'Thanks to your blood sugar diet cookbook', these are words Sarah usually send to me via email. Sarah was able to reclaim her health and her life. She had proven that with determination and the right resources such as this book, it was possible to overcome even the most challenging health conditions.

Globally, type 2 diabetes is becoming more common; it is believed that almost 10% of people globally have this chronic condition. Type 2 diabetes frequently has high blood sugar levels, which can result in a variety of consequences, including nerve damage, renal disease, heart disease, and blindness. For those who already have diabetes as well as those who are at risk of getting it, controlling blood sugar levels is essential.

Diet is one powerful tool for controlling blood sugar levels. Blood sugar levels can be stabilized and post-meal glucose spikes can be avoided with a healthy, balanced diet high in protein, low in carbohydrates, and rich in fiber. A method that has been clinically proved to assist many people control their blood sugar levels and lose weight is the 8-week blood sugar diet.

The 8 Week Blood Sugar eating Cookbook is a thorough manual for adhering to this eating regimen. This cookbook's purpose is to give readers mouthwatering, nutrient-dense dishes that are simple to make and will support their pursuit of a healthy lifestyle. The dishes in this cookbook are specifically adapted to the 8 week blood sugar diet plan and are packed with components that will help regulate blood sugar levels.

There are numerous recipes in the 8 week blood sugar diet cookbook, ranging from breakfast to dinner, snacks, and desserts. The meals in this cookbook are not only healthful but also delectable, making it easier for readers to stick to the diet plan. This cookbook also offers advice on how to plan meals, shop for groceries, and eat out while adhering to the 8-week blood sugar regimen.

The 8 Week Blood Sugar Diet Cookbook is a priceless tool for anyone wishing to reduce their blood sugar levels, whether they have type 2 diabetes or are just trying to get healthier in general. This cookbook's delicious dishes and knowledgeable advice will help you manage your blood sugar levels and reach your health objectives.

What Is The Blood Sugar Diet For 8 Weeks?

The 8 Week Blood Sugar Diet is an eating regimen created to assist people in controlling their blood sugar levels, lowering their chance of developing type 2 diabetes, and also helping them lose weight.

A low-calorie, low-carb, high-protein diet called the "8 Week Blood Sugar Diet" is intended to assist people lose weight quickly while simultaneously stabilizing their blood sugar levels. The diet contains three phases, with particular nutritional requirements and rules for each phase.

Phase 1: The Blood Sugar Diet

The Blood Sugar Diet, which is the first stage of the 8 Week Blood Sugar Diet, consists of 800 calories per day for eight weeks. People are urged to consume a range of low-calorie, low-carbohydrate foods during this phase, including lean protein, non-starchy veggies, and healthy fats. The diet also promotes the consumption of high-fiber foods that help control blood sugar levels, like whole grains and legumes.

Phase 2: The day with the 800 calorie payoff

The 800 calories pay day, which is the second phase of the 8 Week Blood Sugar Diet, lasts for eight weeks. People are advised to consume 800 calories per day during this phase, with the majority of those calories coming from lean proteins and healthy fats. The diet also encourages the eating of nutrient-dense foods including leafy greens, nuts, and seeds and stresses the consumption of high-fiber meals.

Phase 3: The new way of living

The New Way of Life is the eighth and final phase of the 8 Week Blood Sugar Diet. This phase is intended to be a long-term lifestyle adjustment, rather than a short-term eating plan. People are urged to maintain a healthy, balanced diet that includes a range of fruits, vegetables, lean meats, healthy fats, and whole grains during this phase. In order to preserve general health, the diet also urges people to manage their stress, obtain enough sleep, and engage in regular physical activity.

The Advantages of the Blood Sugar Diet for 8 Weeks

Numerous health advantages of the 8 Week Blood Sugar Diet have been demonstrated, including weight loss, better blood sugar regulation, and a lower risk of type 2 diabetes. According to studies, those who follow the 8 Week Blood Sugar Diet can reduce their blood sugar levels dramatically and lose up to 15 kg of weight.

Additionally, the 8 Week Blood Sugar Diet may lower blood pressure, cut inflammation, and raise cholesterol levels, all of which promote general health. The diet is also rather simple to follow, and those who follow the program have access to a broad variety of delicious and nourishing foods.

The 8 Week Blood Sugar Diet, in general, is a successful and scientifically supported program for those wishing to enhance their health, control their blood sugar levels, and accomplish long-term weight loss.

How This Cookbook Can Assist You in Reaching Your Objectives

For persons living with diabetes, managing blood sugar levels is a vital element of preserving their health and lowering the risk of complications connected with this chronic condition. Blood sugar management is greatly influenced by nutrition, however changing one's diet can be challenging for many people. You can use this cookbook, which was created especially for people with diabetes, as a priceless tool to assist you in reaching your health objectives.

Provides Yummy and Healthful Recipes

This cookbook, which is intended for people with diabetes, is brimming with delicious dishes that are also nourishing. These recipes contain components that are high in fiber, low in carbohydrates, and high in protein, and they are designed specifically to help manage blood sugar levels. This cookbook can assist diabetic people feel more motivated and less deprive while adhering to their food plan by offering a selection of delectable meals.

Provides tips for meal planning

This cookbook offers helpful advice on meal planning, assisting you in setting up your meals in advance and maintaining your nutritional objectives. Diabetic patients must plan their meals in order to maintain a regular eating schedule, avoid overeating, and make sure they are eating a balanced diet. This cookbook will offer advice on meal preparation, including how to prepare for snacks and meals when traveling, to make it simpler for you to follow their recommended diet.

Aids Diabetic Patients in Making Knowledgeable Decisions When Eating Out

For diabetics, eating out can be difficult because restaurant food frequently has high carbohydrate counts and hidden sugars. This cookbook is made specifically for people with diabetes to provide them advice on how to make wise decisions when dining out. This can include advice on how to choose healthy selections, read menus, and comprehend how meals at restaurants may affect blood sugar levels.

teaches about wholesome eating practices

This diabetic cookbook features information on sensible eating practices. This contains advice on how to choose nutritious foods, read food labels, comprehend the glycemic index, and regulate portion sizes. This cookbook's material will enable diabetes patients to make better dietary decisions, which will improve blood sugar regulation and general health.

Offers encouragement and support

This cookbook, which was created for diabetic people, provides encouragement and support. Because diabetic-friendly foods are viewed as having a limited variety and taste, many people with diabetes find it difficult to maintain a healthy diet. This cookbook, which is packed with scrumptious and healthy dishes, will provide you the inspiration you need to follow a diet and reach your health objectives.

For those with diabetes who want to control their blood sugar levels and reach their health goals, this cookbook can be a very helpful resource. By giving delicious recipes, meal planning guidance, education on healthy eating habits, and support, this book will help diabetic patients make informed decisions about their diet and maintain long-term health.

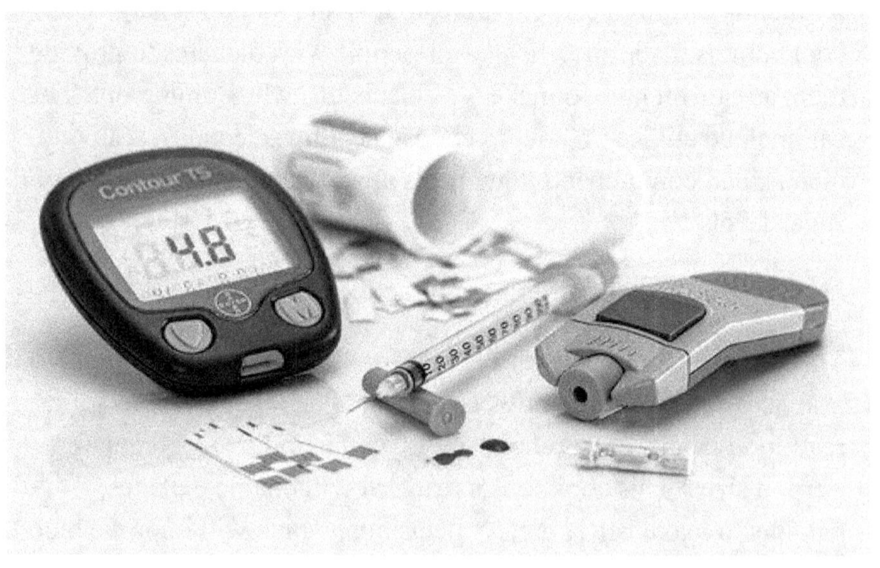

CHAPTER 1

SPECIAL BREAKFAST RECIPES FOR BLOOD SUGAR DIET

For those who have diabetes, a healthy breakfast that is balanced is essential to maintaining their blood sugar levels throughout the day. A breakfast rich in protein and fiber can lessen blood sugar peaks and troughs, enhancing overall health. Here are some delectable, easy-to-make blood sugar diet breakfast recipes that are great for diabetics:

Recipe #1

An omelet with spinach and feta

An omelette with spinach and feta is a delectable, healthy breakfast option that helps regulate blood sugar levels. It is a breakfast that is strong in protein and low in carbs and sugar, making it a great choice for people with diabetes or anybody else seeking to control their blood sugar.

How to prepare for it is as follows:

Ingredients

chopped half a cup of fresh spinach, two enormous embryos

Feta cheese crumbles, 1/4 cup

Olive oil, one tablespoon of pepper, and salt to taste

Ten minutes to prepare

Cooking time: 10 minutes

Cooking Instruction

• Use a whisk to completely beat the eggs in a medium bowl. Use salt and pepper to season food for flavour.

Warm the olive oil in a nonstick frying pan over medium heat.

• Add the spinach, stirring occasionally, and simmer for 1–2 minutes, or until wilted.

Pour the beaten eggs over the spinach in the pan, being careful to spread them evenly.

Sprinkle the feta cheese crumbles on top of the eggs.

The omelette should be cooked for about 4-5 minutes, or until the bottom is golden brown and the sides are starting to set.

• Using a spatula, gently fold the omelette in half.

• Cook the eggs for a further 2 to 3 minutes, or until they are done and the cheese is melted.

• If desired, add more feta cheese and spinach to the omelette before serving.

You can adjust the dish's salt content to your personal preference. You should watch how much sodium you consume. Additionally, this dish includes spinach, a leafy green vegetable that is high in fiber, low in calories and carbohydrates, and ideal for a blood sugar diet. Because of its potent flavor, feta cheese provides flavor and protein, and you only need a minimal amount to achieve the desired results.

Recipe #2

Berry Morning Smoothie

A berry breakfast smoothie is an easy, quick-meal option for breakfast that is great for managing blood sugar. Because it has so many nutrient-dense, low-sugar, and high-fiber ingredients, this smoothie is a terrific choice for anyone seeking to manage their blood sugar levels.

How to prepare for it is as follows:

Ingredients

1/2 cup of frozen mixed berries includes blueberries, strawberries, and raspberries.

Banana half

almond milk without sugar and half a cup of Greek yogurt standard, 1 tbsp. Chia seeds, half a cup.

optional 1 teaspoon of honey

5-minute preparation

Cooking Instruction

The frozen mixed berries, almond milk, Greek yogurt, and chia seeds should all be added to a blender.

• The components should be blended until they are smooth, adding additional almond milk as needed to achieve the desired consistency.

• After tasting the smoothie, if extra sweetness is wanted, add more honey.

• Immediately serve the smoothie, perhaps with some extra berries as a garnish.

Be mindful of your carbohydrate intake and adjust the amount of honey added to this recipe according to your needs. This meal also contains berries, which are an excellent fruit choice for a blood sugar diet because they are high in fiber and low in sugar. Chia seeds and Greek yogurt both boost the amount of protein and healthy fats that can help regulate blood sugar levels. Almond milk offers a low-carbohydrate alternative to dairy milk, making it a wonderful choice for anyone with diabetes or lactose intolerance.

Recipe #3

Almond- and chia-seed-topped porridge

Almond and chia seed porridge is a filling and healthful morning alternative for anyone on a blood sugar diet. Because it is rich in protein, fiber, and healthy fats, this porridge is a terrific choice for people with diabetes or anyone seeking to control their blood sugar levels.

Ingredients

Rolling oats in a cup, adding 1/2 cup of unsweetened almond milk and 1/2 cup of water

1 tablespoon of cinnamon, 1/4 teaspoon of vanilla extract, and 1/4 teaspoon of chia seeds

1 tablespoon of chopped almonds

optional 1 teaspoon of honey

5-minute preparation

For 10 to 15 minutes, cook.

Cooking Instruction

• In a small saucepan, mix the rolled oats, almond milk, water, chia seeds, cinnamon, and vanilla essence.

• Cook the ingredients, stirring occasionally, for 10 to 15 minutes, or until the porridge reaches the desired consistency.

• Once the porridge is cooked through, remove it from the heat and stir in the almonds.

• After tasting the porridge, add additional honey if you prefer it sweeter.

• You can choose to add more almonds on top of the porridge before serving.

Recipes #4

Low-Carb Pancakes

Because they are made with low-glycemic flours like almond and coconut flour and are sweetened with a low-carb sweetener, these pancakes are a great alternative to normal pancakes. How to prepare them is as follows:

Ingredients

1/4 cup coconut flour, 1/2 cup almond flour

1 tablespoon of erythritol or stevia, two low-carb sweeteners,

1/2 a teaspoon of baking powder

1/4 teaspoon of salt

3 eggs

1/4 cup of sugar-free coconut milk

1 teaspoon of coconut oil, 1 teaspoon of liquefied vanilla extract

Ten minutes to prepare

For 10 to 15 minutes, cook.

Cooking Instruction

• In a big mixing bowl, combine the almond flour, coconut flour, low-carb sweetener, baking soda, and salt.

• In a different bowl, combine the eggs, almond milk, melted coconut oil, and vanilla extract.

• To make a smooth batter, mix together the dry ingredients and the wet ones. If the mixture seems too thick, add a bit more almond milk and whisk until the batter is the proper consistency.

• Set a nonstick pan to medium heat on the stovetop. Pour the batter onto the pan once it is hot to make pancakes.

• Cook the pancakes for two to three minutes on each side, or until golden brown and thoroughly cooked.

• Carry out the same procedure with the remaining batter, greasing the pan between each batch as necessary.

Note: Diabetics should be cautious about their carbohydrate intake because low-carb sweetener quantities should be customized to each person's needs. Due to the use of low-glycemic flours and the absence of refined sugar, these pancakes are a great option for a blood sugar diet. The almond and coconut flours provide fiber and good lipids, while the eggs add protein. Almond milk and coconut oil are suitable low-carb alternatives to dairy milk and butter, respectively. Serve these pancakes with fresh fruit and a dollop of plain Greek yogurt for a satisfying and delicious morning.

Recipe #5

Greek Yogurt Parfait

Greek yogurt is a fantastic source of protein, and when paired with fruit and nuts that are high in fiber, it makes the ideal breakfast choice for people with diabetes. Greek yogurt, fresh berries, and chopped almonds should all be layered in a glass or bowl to create a parfait. Pour some honey or maple syrup over top for more sweetness. This nutritious breakfast will keep you full for several hours.

For a blood sugar diet, list the components, the amount of preparation time, and how to make a Greek yogurt parfait.

Ingredients

1 cup of Greek yogurt, plain

a half-cup of mixed berries, including strawberries, blueberries, and raspberries

2 tablespoons of chopped nuts, preferably walnuts or almonds

1 tablespoon of optional honey

5 minutes for preparation

• Combine the Greek yogurt and honey (if using) thoroughly in a small bowl.

• In a glass or bowl, arrange layers of the Greek yogurt mixture, mixed berries, and chopped nuts in the following order: yogurt, berries, nuts.

• Continue until all the ingredients have been used, and then top with a layer of mixed berries and finely chopped nuts.

• You can add more honey if you like.

• Serve right away and delight in!

The blood sugar diet breakfast choice of this Greek yogurt parfait simply takes five minutes to prepare. While the mixed berries and almonds are high in fiber and good fats, the Greek yogurt offers protein. A small amount of sweetness is added by the optional honey without significantly raising blood sugar levels.

Recipe #6

Vegetable-filled omelet

A full and delicious breakfast choice that is ideal for those with diabetes is an omelet with vegetables. In a bowl, whisk together two eggs, season with salt and pepper, and then pour the mixture into a nonstick pan. Add chopped veggies like spinach, mushrooms, onions, and bell peppers. Cook the vegetables and eggs until they are both cooked through. Serve with a piece of whole-wheat toast for a satisfying and full lunch.

Ingredients

two huge eggs

A quarter cup of chopped fresh spinach

1/4 cup feta cheese crumbles

1/fourth cup olive oil

To taste, add salt and pepper.

10 minutes for preparation

Cooking Instruction

The eggs should be cracked into a mixing basin and whisked until completely beaten.

• Stir together the feta cheese and spinach that has been chopped in the bowl.

• Add olive oil to a non-stick skillet and heat over medium-high heat to coat the pan's bottom.

Pour the egg mixture into the skillet after it has warmed up.

• The raw eggs will flow to the edges of the omelette if you use a spatula to gently push the omelette's edges towards the center.

• The omelette should be folded in half and cooked for an additional one to two minutes to ensure that the eggs are properly cooked.

• Season to taste with salt and pepper.

• Serving hot, please.

• Due to its high protein content and low carbohydrate content, this omelette with spinach and feta is a great choice for breakfast on a blood sugar diet. It is simple to make and will provide you all the nutrients you need to start your day off well in only 10 minutes.

Recipe #7

Avocado Toast

Avocado toast is a popular breakfast choice that is excellent for diabetics. Toast a piece of whole-grain bread before covering it with mashed avocado. Add some salt, pepper, and a poached egg for some extra protein. This breakfast is a great choice for people with diabetes because it is high in fiber and good fats.

Note the materials, preparation time, and avocado preparation. For a blood sugar diet, use toast

Ingredients

Whole-grain bread, one slice

ripe avocado, half

A quarter-teaspoon of red pepper flakes

1/fourth cup olive oil

To taste, add salt and pepper.

5 minutes for preparation

Cooking Instruction

• Crisp up the slice of whole-grain bread in the toaster.

• Cut the avocado in half and remove the pit while the bread is browning.

• Scoop the avocado's flesh into a small bowl and mash it with a fork until it is smooth.

• Combine the mashed avocado with the red pepper flakes, olive oil, salt, and pepper.

• Spread the mashed avocado mixture over the toast once it has been lightly toasted.

• If preferred, add more red pepper flakes, salt, and pepper as a garnish.

• Serve right away and delight in!

A nutritious and filling breakfast choice for a blood sugar diet is the avocado toast recipe. The avocado adds healthy fats and vital nutrients, while the whole-grain bread is packed in fiber. This is a wonderful way to start the day because the red pepper flakes give it a spicy kick and can assist to speed up metabolism.

Recipe #8

Chia seed pudding

Chia seeds are a great addition to a blood sugar diet breakfast meal because they are high in protein and fiber. Chia seeds, almond milk, and the sweetener of your choosing should all be combined in a bowl to make chia seed pudding. Mix thoroughly and place in refrigerator for the night. Add fresh berries or chopped nuts to the top in the morning for taste and nutrition.

For a blood sugar diet, list the ingredients, preparation time, and steps for making chia seed pudding.

Ingredients

Chia seeds, 1/4 cup

1 cup of almond milk without sugar

One-half teaspoon of vanilla extract

1 tablespoon of optional honey

14 cup of mixed berries, including strawberries, blueberries, and raspberries

5 minutes for preparation plus 2 hours for cooling

Chia seeds, unsweetened almond milk, vanilla extract, and honey (if used) should all be thoroughly blended in a mixing dish.

• To allow the chia seeds to absorb the liquid, let the mixture sit for 5 minutes.

• To remove any remaining chia seed clumps, stir the mixture once more after 5 minutes.

• Place plastic wrap over the bowl and place in the refrigerator for at least two hours or overnight.

• Stir in the mixed berries when the chia seed pudding has chilled and thickened.

• Enjoy while serving chilled!

This chia seed pudding is a tasty and nourishing breakfast choice for blood sugar diets that is rich in fiber, healthy fats, and necessary nutrients. This filling breakfast is an excellent way to start the day because chia seeds are a fantastic source of plant-based protein. The mixed berries' natural sweetness and low sugar content help to maintain stable blood sugar levels. For a quick and simple breakfast on the run, the pudding can be prepared in advance and kept in the refrigerator.

Recipe #9

Overnight Oats

A quick and practical breakfast option that can be made ahead of time is overnight oats. Rolling oats, almond milk, Greek yogurt, and a sweetener of your choosing should all be combined in a jar to make overnight oats. Place it in the refrigerator overnight and then add the chopped nuts, seeds, and fresh fruit. Add more fruit to the top in the morning for taste and nutrition.

Ingredients

Rolling oats in a cup, half

Unsweetened almond milk in 1/2 cup

Cinnamon, 1/4 teaspoon

Vanilla extract, half a teaspoon

Chia seeds, 1 tbsp

Fresh blueberries, raspberries, and strawberries, 1/4 cup

1-tablespoon worth of chopped nuts (walnuts, pecans, almonds)

1 teaspoon of optional honey

5 minutes to prepare

• Combine the rolled oats, almond milk without added sugar, cinnamon, vanilla essence, and chia seeds in a bowl or container. Mix thoroughly.

• Sprinkle chopped nuts and fresh berries over the oat mixture. Adding honey is optional.

• Place the bowl or jar in the fridge for at least 6 to 8 hours.

• Stir the oats in the morning and, if necessary, add extra almond milk to change the consistency. Offer chilled.

Note: Individual needs should be considered when adjusting the amount of honey added to this recipe and diabetic individuals should be cautious about their carbohydrate intake. This recipe also contains nutrient-dense components that are high in fiber and protein, low in sugar, and can help control blood sugar levels.

Recipes #10

Pancakes

These pancakes are a terrific substitute for regular pancakes since they are produced with low-glycemic flours like almond and coconut flour and are sweetened with a low-carb sweetener. Here's how to get them ready:

Ingredients

Almond flour, half a cup

coconut flour, 1/4 cup

1 tablespoon of a low-carb sweetener, such as erythritol or stevia

Baking powder, half a teaspoon

Salt, 1/4 teaspoon

3 eggs

1/4 cup of almond milk without sugar

1 tablespoon of coconut oil, melted

Vanilla extract, half a teaspoon

10 minutes for preparation

Cook for 10 to 15 minutes.

Cooking Instruction

• Combine the almond flour, coconut flour, low-carb sweetener, baking soda, and salt in a sizable mixing basin.

• Combine the eggs, almond milk, melted coconut oil, and vanilla extract in a another bowl.

• While whisking, combine the wet components with the dry ones to create a smooth batter. Add a little more almond milk if the mixture looks too thick and stir until the batter is the right consistency.

• Put a nonstick pan on the stovetop at medium heat. When the pan is heated, pour the batter onto it to create pancakes.

• Cook the pancakes until golden brown and cooked through, about 2-3 minutes per side.

• Repeat with the remaining batter, lubricating the pan as necessary in between each batch.

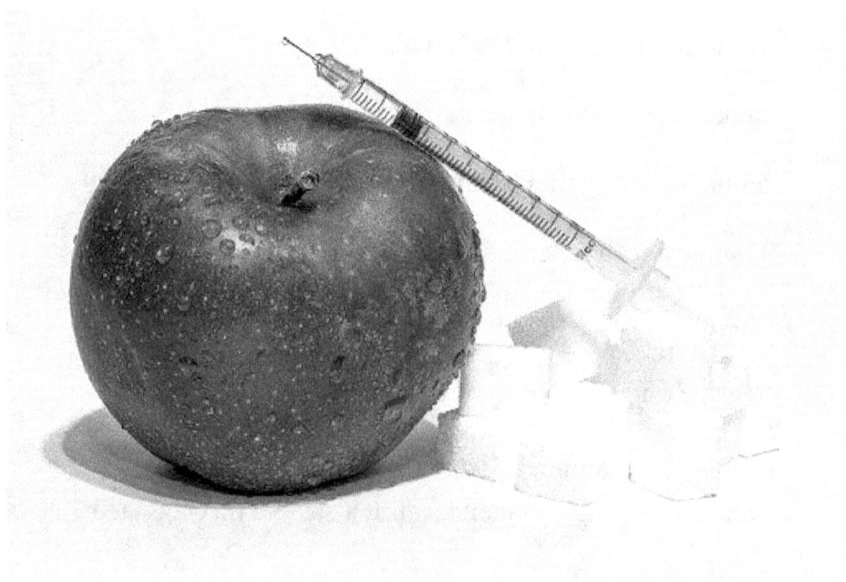

CHAPTER 2

LUNCH RECIPES THAT ARE

HEALTHY

For anyone on a blood sugar diet, lunch is a crucial meal. To assist control blood sugar levels and keep you feeling full and content throughout the afternoon, it's crucial to have a balanced combination of protein, healthy fats, and low-glycemic carbohydrates.

These delectable lunch ideas are ideal for a blood sugar diet book:

Recipe 1

Stir-fried chicken with vegetables

Ingredients

Olive oil, 1 tbsp

2 cups of mixed vegetables (such as broccoli, bell peppers, and mushrooms) and 1 pound of boneless, skinless chicken breast

1 minced garlic clove

Low-sodium soy sauce, 1 tbsp

Cornstarch, 1 tablespoon

one-fourth cup of chicken broth

• In a big skillet over medium-high heat, warm the olive oil.

• Stir in the chicken breast slices and cook for 3 to 4 minutes, or until browned all over.

• Stir-fry the garlic and mixed vegetables for a further 2–3 minutes in the skillet.

• Combine the soy sauce, cornstarch, and chicken broth in a small bowl.

Stir the sauce into the skillet after adding it.

• Cook the sauce for a further one to two minutes, or until it has thickened.

• Immediately serve the stir-fry, if desired garnished with sesame seeds or thinly sliced scallions.

Recipe 2

Salad of lentils and roasted vegetables

Ingredients

1 cup of washed and drained dried lentils

2 cups of various veggies, diced into bite-sized pieces (such as sweet potatoes, carrots, and red onions).

Olive oil, 1 tbsp

Baby spinach leaves in 2 cups

1/4 cup of feta cheese crumbles

Balsamic vinegar, two tablespoons

1/fourth cup of Dijon mustard

1 minced garlic clove

pepper and salt as desired

Cooking Instruction

Set the oven's temperature to 400 °F.

On a baking sheet, spread the chopped vegetables and sprinkle with olive oil. Add salt and pepper to taste.

Vegetables should be roasted for 20 to 25 minutes, or until they are soft and caramelized.

• Cook the lentils per the directions on the package while the vegetables are roasting.

• Combine the balsamic vinegar, Dijon mustard, garlic, salt, and pepper in a small bowl.

• Combine the cooked lentils, roasted veggies, and young spinach leaves in a big bowl.

• Dress the salad with the balsamic vinegar and toss to mix.

• Just before serving, garnish the salad with feta cheese crumbles.

Recipe 3

Lettuce Wraps With Turkey And Avocado

Ingredients

1 pound of turkey meat

Olive oil, 1 tbsp

1 minced garlic clove

Chili powder, 1/4 teaspoon

pepper and salt as desired

4 big leaves of lettuce

1 sliced avocado

1/4 cup freshly chopped cilantro

wedges sliced from 1 lime

Cooking Instruction

• In a big skillet over medium-high heat, warm the olive oil.

• Add the ground turkey and heat it through, breaking it up with a spatula as it cooks.

Stir in the minced garlic, chili powder, salt, and pepper after adding them to the skillet.

Spoon the cooked turkey mixture onto each lettuce leaf after arranging the lettuce leaves on a platter.

Sliced avocado, chopped cilantro, and a squeeze of lime juice should be placed on top of each lettuce wrap.

• Immediately serve the lettuce wraps with more lime wedges on the side, if preferred.

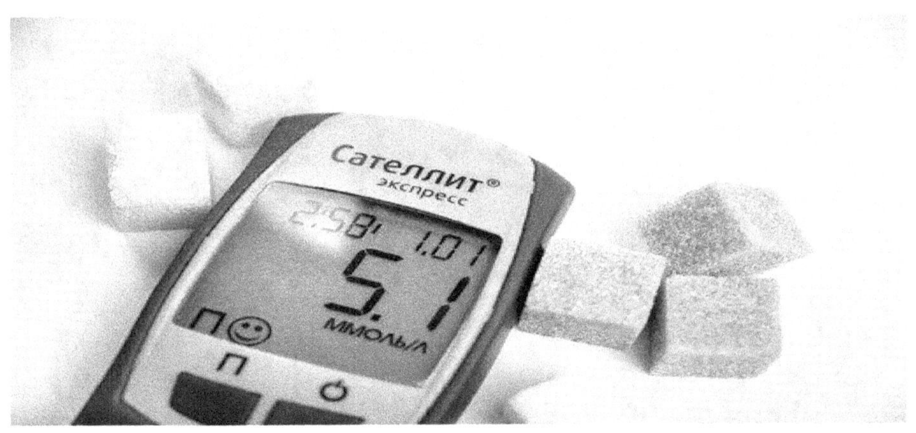

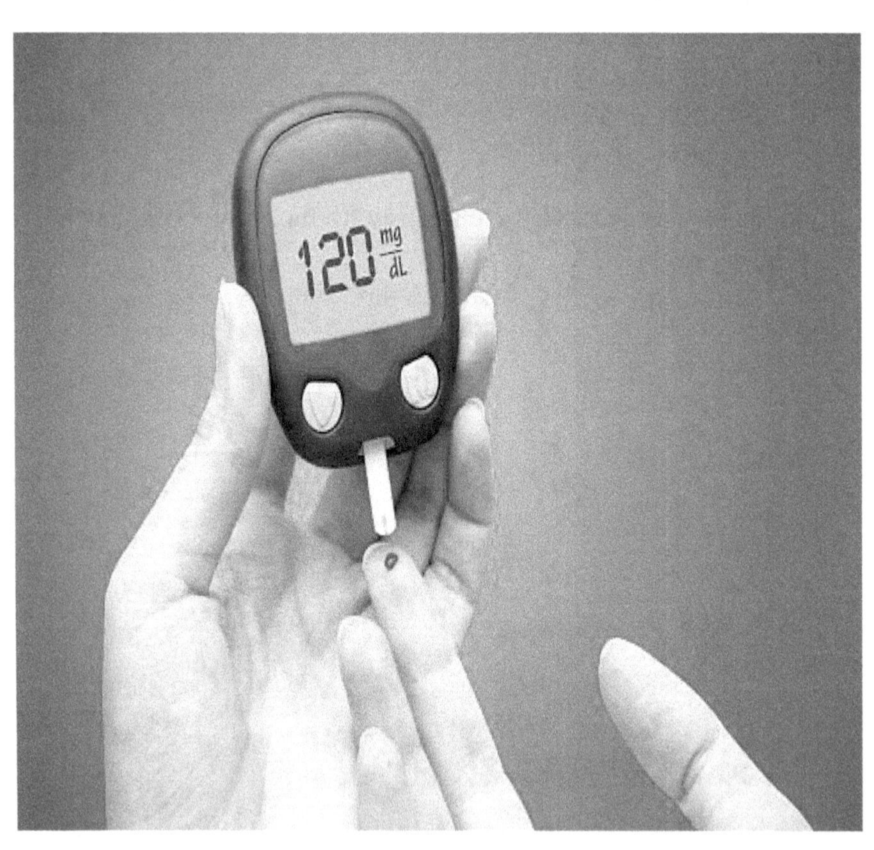

CHAPTER 3

HEALTHY AND DELECTABLE

DINNER RECIPES

Dinner is a crucial meal of the day, therefore it's crucial to pick components that can keep your blood sugar levels in a healthy range.

Here are some dinner recipes that are delectable and healthful and would be a wonderful addition to your blood sugar diet:

Recipe 1

Steak On The Grill With Chimichurri Sauce

For people on a blood sugar diet, grilled steak with chimichurri sauce makes a delightful and nutritious supper choice. Traditional Argentinean sauces like chimichurri are created with fresh herbs, garlic, vinegar, and olive oil. How to prepare grilled steak with chimichurri sauce is as follows:

Ingredients

2 beef steaks (ribeye or sirloin)

Pepper and salt

14 cup chopped fresh parsley

a third of a clove of minced garlic and 1/4 cup fresh cilantro

Red wine vinegar, 1/4 cup

Olive oil, 1/4 cup

optional 1/2 tsp red pepper flakes

Cooking Instruction

• Set the grill to a high heat.

• Liberally sprinkle salt and pepper on both sides of the steaks.

Depending on how well done you prefer your steak, place the steaks on the grill and cook for 4-5 minutes per side.

• Make the chimichurri sauce and set it aside while the steaks are cooking. Combine the parsley, cilantro, garlic, red wine vinegar, extra virgin olive oil, and red pepper flakes (if using) in a small bowl.

• When the steaks are done to your preference, take them from the grill and give them a few minutes to rest.

• Serve the steaks immediately after spooning the chimichurri sauce over them.

This delectable and nutritious steak dish is grilled and served with chimichurri sauce. It is ideal for a blood sugar diet. The steak offers a fantastic source of protein, and the chimichurri sauce, with its fresh herbs and nutritious olive oil, adds flavor and nutrition. For a filling and complete supper, serve with a side of roasted vegetables or a mixed green salad.

Recipe 2

Salmon baked in herb butter

For individuals on a blood sugar diet, baked salmon with herbed butter is a delectable and healthful dinner option. Here's how to prepare this tasty and healthy dish:

Ingredients

4 salmon fillets, each 6 ounces

Pepper and salt

14 cup softened unsalted butter

two tablespoons of freshly chopped parsley and dill

1 tablespoon lemon juice, fresh

1 minced garlic clove

Cooking Instruction

• Set your oven to 375 degrees.

• Liberally salt and pepper the salmon fillets on both sides.

• Combine the butter that has been softened with the parsley, dill, lemon juice, and garlic in a small bowl. Blend thoroughly.

• Salmon fillets should be put on a baking pan covered with parchment paper.

Each salmon fillet should have the herbed butter mixture spread on top of it.

• Bake the salmon for 12 to 15 minutes in a preheated oven, or until it is cooked through and flakes readily with a fork.

• Take the salmon out of the oven and give it some time to rest before serving.

A delicious and nutritious dinner choice that is ideal for a blood sugar diet is baked salmon with herbed butter. The herbed butter, which contains fresh herbs and excellent fats from butter, enhances flavor and nutrition while the salmon is a fantastic amount of protein and omega-3 fatty acids. For a filling and complete supper, serve with a side of roasted vegetables or a mixed green salad.

Recipe 3

Beef Stew in the Slow Cooker

A rich and comfortable meal choice for folks on a blood sugar diet is slow cooker beef stew. Here's how to prepare this tasty and healthy dish:

Ingredients

2 pounds of cubed beef stew meat

Pepper and salt

2/TBS of olive oil

one sliced onion

3 minced garlic cloves

3 chopped carrots, 3 chopped celery stalks, and 1 cup of beef broth

1 glass red wine

1.5 tbsp tomato paste

1 bay leaf, 2

Dry thyme, 1 teaspoon

1 teaspoon dried rosemary

1 pound of chopped potatoes

Frozen peas, 1 cup

Cooking Instruction

• Sprinkle salt and pepper over the beef stew meat on all sides.

• In a big skillet over medium-high heat, warm the olive oil. When browned, add the beef stew meat and cook for 3–4 minutes on each side. Enter the slow cooker with the beef.

• Cook the carrots, celery, onion, and garlic in the same skillet for 3 to 4 minutes, or until tender. the slow cooker with the vegetables.

• Fill the slow cooker with the beef broth, red wine, tomato paste, bay leaves, thyme, and rosemary. To blend, stir.

• Cook the beef in the slow cooker with the lid on for 6 to 8 hours on low, or until it is tender.

• Place the peas and potatoes in the slow cooker, stirring to incorporate. The potatoes should be soft after another 30 to 60 minutes of cooking with the cover on.

• Before serving, take the bay leaves out of the stew.

For a tasty and nutritious dinner choice that is ideal for a blood sugar diet, try this slow cooker beef stew. The vegetables contribute fiber and nutrients, and the beef serves as a solid source of protein. For a complete and filling dinner, serve with a side of whole grain bread or a mixed green salad.

Recipe 4

Turkey Avocado Chili

A tasty and nutritious dinner option for folks on a blood sugar diet is turkey chili with avocado. Here's how to prepare this tasty and healthy dish:

Ingredients

1 pound of turkey meat

1 diced onion, 3 minced garlic cloves

a red bell pepper, a green bell pepper, and a jalapeño pepper, all sliced up

1.5 tbsp cumin powder

2 teaspoons cumin powder

1 teaspoon paprika

Cayenne pepper, 1/2 tsp

12 teaspoon salt

two (15 oz) cans shredded tomatoes

1 can (15 oz) washed and drained kidney beans

1 can (15 oz) washed and drained black beans

0.5 cups of water

1 diced avocado

2 tbsp freshly chopped cilantro

Cooking Instruction

• Place a large skillet over high heat. After adding, sauté the ground turkey for 5–6 minutes, or until browned. Put the turkey in the slow cooker.

• Fill the slow cooker with the onion, garlic, bell peppers, jalapenos, chili powder, cumin, paprika, cayenne pepper, and salt. To blend, stir.

• Fill the slow cooker with water, kidney beans, black beans, and diced tomatoes. To blend, stir.

• Cook the food in the slow cooker with the lid on for 6 to 8 hours on low, or until the veggies are soft and the flavors are well-balanced.

• Top the hot turkey chili with diced avocado and cilantro before serving.

An excellent and savory dinner choice that is ideal for a blood sugar diet is this turkey chili with avocado. The beans and vegetables contribute fiber and nutrients, while the ground turkey offers a decent amount of protein. The avocado gives the chili healthful lipids and a creamy mouthfeel. For a complete and filling dinner, serve with a side of whole grain crackers or a mixed green salad.

Recipe 5

Roasted vegetables and grilled chicken

The meal's roasted veggies and grilled chicken, both excellent sources of protein, add fiber and nutrients.

Chicken breasts should be marinated for a few hours in olive oil, garlic, and lemon juice to make this dish. Cook the chicken on the grill until it is fully cooked, then serve it with roasted veggies such bell peppers, zucchini, and eggplant. Use herbs and spices like oregano, rosemary, and thyme to season food.

Recipe 6

Turkey Meatballs Over 6 Zucchini Noodles

Zoodles, also known as zucchini noodles, are a fantastic low-carb substitute for pasta. Combine ground turkey with chopped onions, garlic, parsley, and egg to make turkey meatballs. Make into tiny balls, then bake in the oven until done. Serve the meatballs with zucchini noodles that have been tossed in a pan with garlic, olive oil, and cherry tomatoes. Add fresh herbs and Parmesan cheese on top.

Recipe 7

Fried rice with cauliflower

Rice made from cauliflower is a fantastic low-carb substitute for regular rice. Process cauliflower florets in a food processor until they resemble rice to make cauliflower fried rice. Cook the cauliflower rice while adding vegetables like carrots, peas, and onions. When adding protein, season with soy sauce and ginger and add cooked chicken or shrimp.

Recipe 8

Salmon with Asparagus Baked

Salmon is a fantastic source of protein and omega-3 fatty acids. Salmon fillets should be seasoned with herbs like dill and thyme to make this dish. Cook in the oven until fully done. Serve with side salads of mixed greens dressed with a mild vinaigrette and roasted asparagus.

Recipe 9

Vegetable and Lentil Soup

Due to their high protein and dietary fiber content, lentils are a fantastic complement to a blood sugar diet. In order to cook lentil and vegetable soup, soften chopped celery, onions, and carrots in olive oil. Lentils, chicken or vegetable broth, and chopped spinach, tomatoes, and zucchini are all recommended. Till the lentils are cooked, simmer. Use herbs like rosemary and thyme to season.

These dinner recipes are scrumptious, healthy, and simple to make. You may maintain a healthy blood sugar level and enhance your general health by including low-carbohydrate, low-sugar, and high-fiber foods in your meals.

Recipe 10

Grilled Steak with Chimichurri Sauce

For people on a blood sugar diet, grilled steak with chimichurri sauce makes a delightful and nutritious supper choice. Traditional Argentinean sauces like chimichurri are created with fresh herbs, garlic, vinegar, and olive oil. How to prepare grilled steak with chimichurri sauce is as follows:

Ingredients

2 beef steaks (ribeye or sirloin)

Pepper and salt

3 garlic cloves, minced, along with 1/4 cup fresh parsley and 1/4 cup fresh cilantro.

Red wine vinegar, 1/4 cup

Olive oil, 1/4 cup

optional 1/2 tsp red pepper flakes

Cooking Instruction

• Set the grill to a high heat.

• Liberally sprinkle salt and pepper on both sides of the steaks.

Depending on how well done you prefer your steak, place the steaks on the grill and cook for 4-5 minutes per side.

• Make the chimichurri sauce and set it aside while the steaks are cooking. Combine the parsley, cilantro, garlic, red wine vinegar, extra virgin olive oil, and red pepper flakes (if using) in a small bowl.

• When the steaks are done to your preference, take them from the grill and give them a few minutes to rest.

• Serve the steaks immediately after spooning the chimichurri sauce over them.

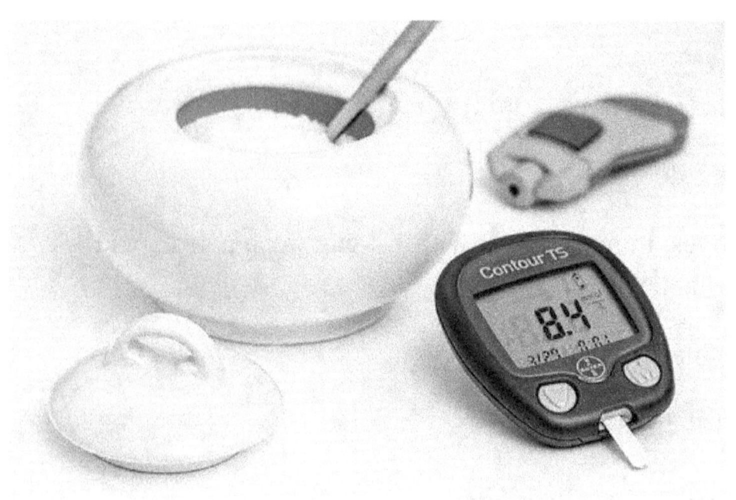

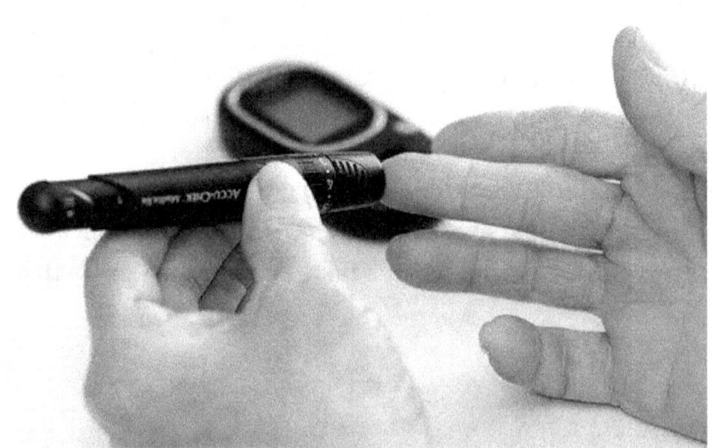

CHAPTER 4

In order to control blood sugar levels throughout the day and avoid overeating at meals, snacks can be a crucial component of a blood sugar diet.

Here are some recipes for nutritious and delectable snacks that are ideal for a blood sugar diet:

Recipe 1

Roasted Chickpeas

Ingredients

1 cup of roasted chickpeas

1 can (15 oz) washed and drained chickpeas

1 tablespoon of olive oil

1 teaspoon chili powder

12 teaspoon of garlic powder

14 teaspoon salt

Cooking Instruction

Set the oven's temperature to 400 °F.

The chickpeas should be rinsed, drained, and dried with paper towels.

• Combine the chickpeas in a bowl with the salt, garlic powder, chili powder, and olive oil.

• On a baking sheet, distribute the chickpeas in a single layer.

• Roast, tossing periodically, for 25 to 30 minutes or until crisp and golden brown.

• Servable at room temperature or warm.

Recipe 2

Veggie and Hummus Snack Plate

Ingredients

a variety of fresh vegetables (including carrot sticks, bell pepper strips, cucumber slices, and cherry tomatoes)

14 cup of hummus

1 tbsp. freshly chopped parsley

Cooking Instruction

The vegetables should be washed, cut into slices, and placed on a platter.

Place a small dish of hummus on the plate after ladling some into it.

Add some chopped parsley to the hummus and vegetables.

as a wholesome and gratifying snack.

Recipe 3

Apple And Almond Butter Sandwiches

Ingredients

Round slices of one apple

2/butter almonds

1/4 cup chopped almonds

1/8 teaspoon cinnamon

Cooking Instruction

• Remove the apple's core before cutting it into rounds.

Each apple round should have almond butter applied to one side.

• Top the almond butter with cinnamon and sliced almonds.

• To make a sandwich, add another apple round on top.

• Either serve right away or cover with plastic wrap and store in the fridge.

Recipe 4

Greek yogurt and berry parfait.

Ingredients

Greek yogurt, plain, in 1/2 cup

14 cup of mixed berries, including strawberries, blueberries, and raspberries

chopped walnuts, 1 tablespoon

1 teaspoon of honey

Cooking Instruction

• Combine the Greek yogurt and honey in a small bowl.

In a glass or small bowl, arrange the yogurt mixture, berries, and chopped walnuts.Either serve right now or cover and chill for later.

All of these nutritious, simple snack ideas are ideal for a blood sugar diet. They offer a balanced serving of protein, fiber, and healthy fats that keep blood sugar levels stable and your hunger pangs at bay between meals.

<h1 align="center">Recipe 5</h1>

Hummus with Roasted Garlic

Burnt Garlic A blood sugar diet is ideal for hummus because it is a tasty and healthful snack. It is a fantastic source of protein, fiber, and healthy fats and is made with chickpeas, tahini, lemon juice, and roasted garlic. This is how to do it:

Ingredients

1 can (15 oz) washed and drained chickpeas

Tahini, 14 cup

1-2 roasted garlic cloves*, 3 tablespoons of lemon juice

14 teaspoon cumin

14 teaspoon paprika

14 teaspoon salt

14 cup of water

2/TBS of olive oil

Cooking Instruction

Set the oven's temperature to 400 °F.

• Slice off the top of a head of garlic, cover with foil, spray with olive oil, and roast for 30-35 minutes, or until tender and aromatic.

The chickpeas should be rinsed, drained, and dried with paper towels.

• Combine the chickpeas, tahini, roasted garlic, lemon juice, cumin, paprika, and salt in a food processor.

• Pulse the ingredients until it is creamy and smooth.

• Slowly add the water and olive oil to the food processor while it is running until the hummus is the right consistency.

• Taste the food, then season as necessary.

• You can either serve the hummus right away with extra olive oil and paprika on top, or you can keep it in the fridge for up to a week in an airtight container.

• Set the oven to 400°F and roast the garlic there. A head of garlic should have the top cut off, be drizzled with oil, wrapped in foil, and roasted for 30 to 35 minutes, or until tender and aromatic. Before adding in the hummus, allow to cool.

Recipe 6

Almonds with spices

A delicious and nutritious snack that is ideal for a blood sugar diet is spiced almonds. They are tasty and nutritious, and they are simple to create. How to manufacture them is as follows:

Ingredients

2 cups of almonds, raw

1 tablespoon of olive oil

1 tablespoon honey, 2 teaspoons ground cinnamon

1/2 tsp. of ginger powder

Ground nutmeg, 1/4 teaspoon

14 teaspoon salt

Recipe Directions

Set the oven's temperature to 350 °F.

• Combine the raw almonds, honey, and olive oil in a sizable bowl. Stir the almonds thoroughly to coat them.

• Combine the salt, nutmeg, cinnamon, and ginger in a small bowl.

• After the almonds are well covered, sprinkle the spice mixture over them and stir.

• Arrange the almonds on a baking sheet that has been lined with parchment paper in a single layer.

• Bake the almonds for 10 to 12 minutes, or until aromatic and gently browned.

Prior to serving, let the almonds cool on the baking pan for a few minutes.

• You can keep any leftover spiced almonds at room temperature for up to a week in an airtight container.

Protein, fiber, healthy fats, and essential vitamins and minerals like vitamin E, magnesium, and potassium are all found in abundance in spiced almonds. They provide a delicious and healthy between-meal snack that can support stable blood sugar levels.

Recipe 7

Apple with peanut butter

A traditional snack that is both tasty and healthy, apple and peanut butter is a great option for a blood sugar diet. While peanut butter is an excellent source of protein and healthy fats, apples are a good supply of fiber, vitamins, and antioxidants. Here is how to prepare this easy and filling snack:

Ingredients

1 sliced medium apple

Natural peanut butter, 2 tablespoons

Cooking Instruction

• Wash the apple and cut it into little wedges.

• Place a small bowl with the peanut butter in it.

Enjoy dipping the apple slices in the peanut butter!

Alternatively, if you like, you can use almond or cashew butter in place of peanut butter and spread it with a knife onto the apple slices. You may top this snack with ingredients like sliced banana, chia seeds, or ground almonds to make it even more full and healthy. To keep track of the calories and carbohydrates in this snack, make sure to measure the peanut butter and toppings.

Recipe 8

guacamole with veggie sticks. is a tasty and wholesome snack that is ideal for a blood sugar diet. While vegetables like carrots, celery, and cucumber are low in calories and high in fiber and minerals, avocados are a terrific source of healthy fats, fiber, and potassium. Here's how to prepare this quick and tasty snack:

Ingredients

Two mature avocados

1 sliced small tomato

1/4 diced red onion

1 jalapeño pepper, minced after being seeded

1 minced garlic clove

1 juiced lime

To taste, add salt and pepper.

Various vegetable sticks, including cucumber, celery, and carrots

Cut the avocados in half, scoop out the meat into a basin after removing the pit.

• Using a fork, mash the avocado until it is mostly smooth but still has a few small bits.

• Stir together the minced garlic, red onion, jalapeño pepper, and tomato in the bowl after adding them.

• Give the guacamole another swirl after adding the juice of one lime.

• Add salt and pepper to taste and season the guacamole.

• Provide a variety of veggie sticks for dipping along with the guacamole.

While savoring the creamy, savory pleasure of guacamole, this snack is a terrific way to get your daily serving of vegetables. Additionally, it's an excellent source of fiber, healthful fats, and essential vitamins and minerals including potassium and vitamin C. To keep an eye on the calories and carbohydrates in this snack, just be sure to measure out the guacamole and veggie sticks.

CHAPTER 5

RECIPES FOR SWEETS

A blood sugar diet does not need complete dessert abstinence! You can enjoy a variety of delectable and healthful dessert recipes while still managing your blood sugar levels. Here are some suggestions for tasty and healthy desserts:

Recipe 1

Crispy Mixed Berry

A delicious and nutritious dessert that is ideal for blood sugar dieters is mixed berry crisp. It is covered in a crispy, oat-filled topping and brimming with luscious berries. A recipe for Mixed Berry Crisp is given below:

Ingredients

strawberries, blueberries, and raspberries made up of 4 cups

1/3 cup honey and 1/4 cup cornstarch

one teaspoon of lemon juice

Old-fashioned rolled oats, 1/2 cup

14 cup almond meal

chopped walnuts, 1/4 cup

a quarter cup of melted coconut oil

1/four teaspoons of cinnamon

A dash of salt

Cooking Instruction

• Set the oven to 375 degrees.

• Combine the berries, honey, cornstarch, and lemon juice in a sizable mixing basin. Blend thoroughly.

• The berry mixture should be added to an 8x8 baking dish.

• Combine the oats, almond flour, chopped walnuts, melted coconut oil, cinnamon, and salt in a different mixing dish. Mix until the dough is crumbly and the ingredients are thoroughly incorporated.

• Over the berry mixture, evenly distribute the oat mixture.

• Place the preheated oven on the middle rack and bake the mixed berry crisp for 25 to 30 minutes, or until the topping is golden brown and the berries are bubbling.

• Take the dish out of the oven and let it cool before serving.

Enjoy this mouthwatering Mixed Berry Crisp as a delightful and healthful dessert that won't cause a blood sugar surge.

Recipe 2

Lemon And Blueberry Cheesecake

Lemon and Blueberry Cheesecake Bars are a delicious and filling dessert that are ideal for blood sugar diet followers. This recipe makes a low-carb, gluten-free crust out of almond flour and Swerve sweetener, which is then filled with a creamy, lemony cheesecake filling and topped with sweet blueberry sauce.

The recipe for these Lemon and Blueberry Cheesecake Bars is as follows:

Ingredients

Almond flour, two cups

Swerve sweetener, 1/4 cup

14 teaspoon of salt

14 cup of melted butter

When filling:

16 ounces of softened cream cheese

Swerve sweetener, half a cup

two huge eggs

10 grams of lemon zest

Lemon juice, two tablespoons

Regarding the berry sauce:

2 cups blueberries, either fresh or frozen

Swerve sweetener, 1/4 cup

water in 2 tablespoons

one teaspoon of lemon juice

Cooking Instruction

Set the oven's temperature to 350 °F.

• Place parchment paper on the bottom of an 8x8-inch baking pan.

• In a medium mixing bowl, combine the almond flour, Swerve sweetener, and salt to make the crust. When the mixture is crumbly, add the melted butter and stir.

• Firmly press the crust mixture into the prepared baking dish's bottom. After 10 minutes of baking, take from the oven and place on a cooling rack.

• In a sizable mixing basin, combine the cream cheese and Swerve sweetener and beat until combined. Beat in the eggs, lemon juice, and zest after adding them.

• Over the cooled crust, pour the filling mixture.

• In a small saucepan, combine the blueberries, Swerve sweetener, water, and lemon juice to produce the blueberry sauce. Stirring occasionally, bring the mixture to a boil, then lower the heat and simmer for 10 to 15 minutes, or until the sauce has thickened.

Over the cheesecake filling, drizzle the blueberry sauce.

• Bake the cheesecake bars for 30-35 minutes, or until the filling has set, in a preheated oven.

• Take out of the oven, let cool to room temperature, then chill for at least two hours in the refrigerator before slicing and serving.

Take pleasure in these delectable Lemon and Blueberry Cheesecake Bars as a filling and healthful treat that won't cause a blood sugar surge.

Recipe 3

Brownies with Coconut Flour

For individuals on a blood sugar diet, coconut flour brownies are a delectable and healthy dessert alternative. These low-carb, gluten-free, and grain-free brownies nonetheless have a deep, chocolatey flavor. Coconut flour, which has a little coconut taste, is used in place of regular wheat flour to reduce the amount of carbohydrates in the brownies. The recipe for Coconut Flour Brownies is as follows:

Ingredients

a half-cup of coconut flour

a half-cup of cocoa powder

A half-teaspoon of baking powder

14 teaspoon of salt

Melted 1/2 cup coconut oil

Swerve sweetener, half a cup

Four big eggs

Vanilla extract, 1 teaspoon

Cooking Instruction

Set the oven's temperature to 350 °F. Use coconut oil to grease an 8x8-inch baking dish.

• Combine the coconut flour, cocoa powder, baking soda, and salt in a medium mixing basin.

• Whisk the melted coconut oil and Swerve sweetener thoroughly in a large mixing dish.

• Stir the coconut oil mixture well after adding the eggs and vanilla essence.

• Stir the batter until it is smooth after adding the dry ingredients to the wet ones.

• Spoon the batter into the prepared baking dish, then use a spatula to smooth the surface.

• Bake for 20 to 25 minutes in a preheated oven, or until a toothpick inserted in the center of the brownies comes out clean.

• Before slicing and serving, let the brownies cool in the pan for at least 10 minutes.

Enjoy these tasty Coconut Flour Brownies as a guilt-free treat that won't cause your blood sugar to surge.

Recipe 4

Berry Sorbet

A dessert for a blood sugar diet, this tasty and reviving sorbet is reduced in calories and sugar. This is how to do it:

Ingredients

2 cups of frozen mixed berries, including blueberries, raspberries, and strawberries

14 cup of water

1 tablespoon maple syrup or honey (optional)

1/2 lemon juice

Cooking Instruction

• Use a food processor or blender to combine the frozen berries.

• Include the water, lemon juice, and honey or maple syrup (if using).

• Blend the mixture until it's creamy and smooth.

• Serve the sorbet right away by scooping it into dishes or glasses.

Recipe 5

Avocado and Chocolate Pudding

This creamy, thick pudding is a powerhouse of fiber, antioxidants, and good fats. This is how to do it:

Ingredients

Two mature avocados

Unsweetened cocoa powder, 1/4 cup

1/4 cup maple syrup or honey

1/4 cup of almond milk without sugar

Vanilla extract, 1 teaspoon

Cooking Instruction

• Halve the avocados, scoop out the pit, and add the flesh to a food processor or blender.

• Include the almond milk, vanilla essence, honey or maple syrup, and chocolate powder.

• Process the mixture until it is creamy and smooth.

• Pour the pudding into dishes or glasses and chill for at least 30 minutes in the fridge.

• Top the chilled pudding with whipped coconut cream, sliced berries, or chopped almonds as desired.

Recipe 6

Apples Baked

This dish is a healthy take on traditional apple pie that is warm and cozy. This is how to do it:

Ingredients

4 large apples

1 cup of raisins

chopped walnuts, 1/4 cup

1 tablespoon of maple syrup or honey

1 teaspoon of cinnamon

14 teaspoon nutmeg

14 cup of water

Recipe Directions

• Set the oven to 375 degrees.

• After washing the apples, remove the stem and core by cutting off the top of each apple.

• Combine the raisins, walnuts, honey or maple syrup, cinnamon, and nutmeg in a small bowl.

• Tightly pack the mixture into the center of each apple.

• Put the apples in a baking dish and fill the bottom of the dish with water.

The apples should be baked for 30 to 40 minutes, or until they are soft and the filling has caramelized.

• Top the warm apples with whipped cream or Greek yogurt (if desired) and serve immediately.

These dessert recipes are only a sample of the many mouthwatering and nutritious options that may be included in a blood sugar diet. To control your blood sugar levels, keep an eye on the calories and carbs in each dish and enjoy them in moderation.

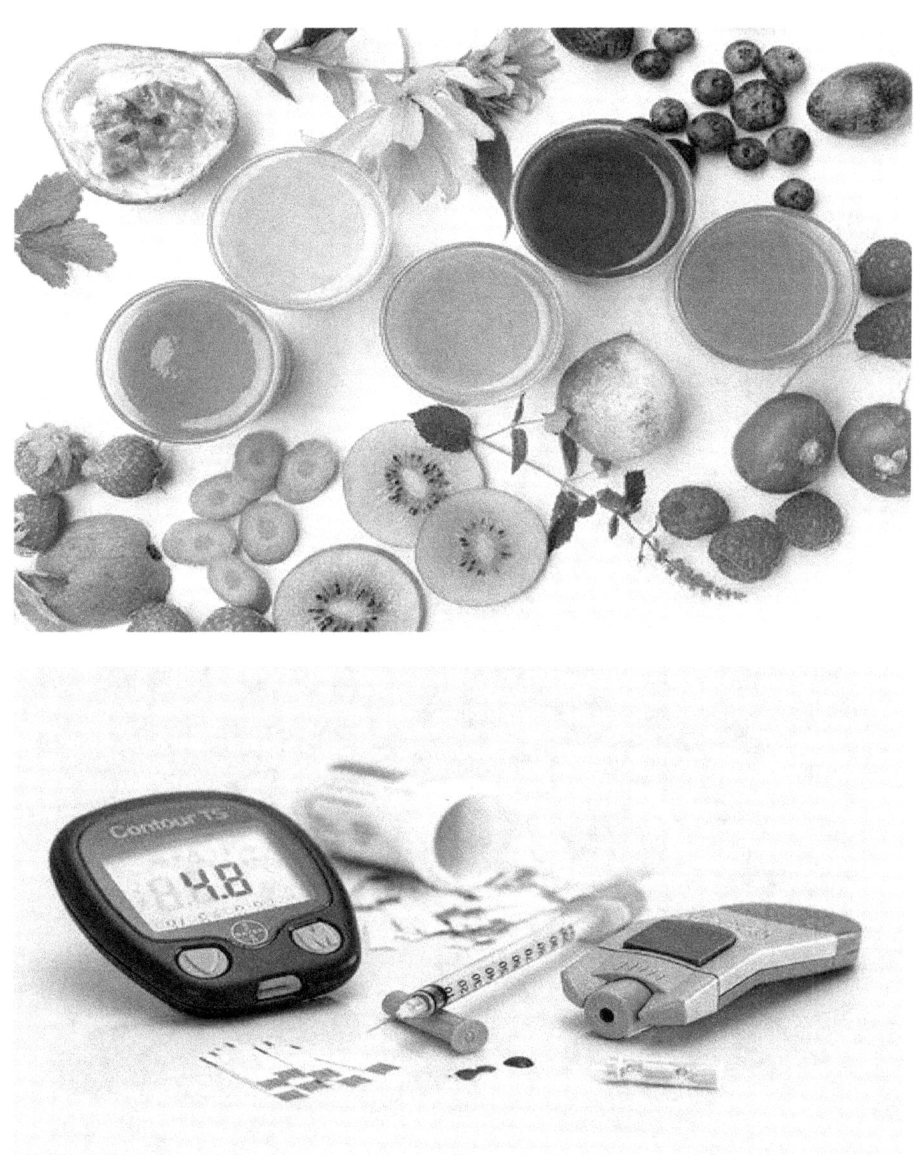

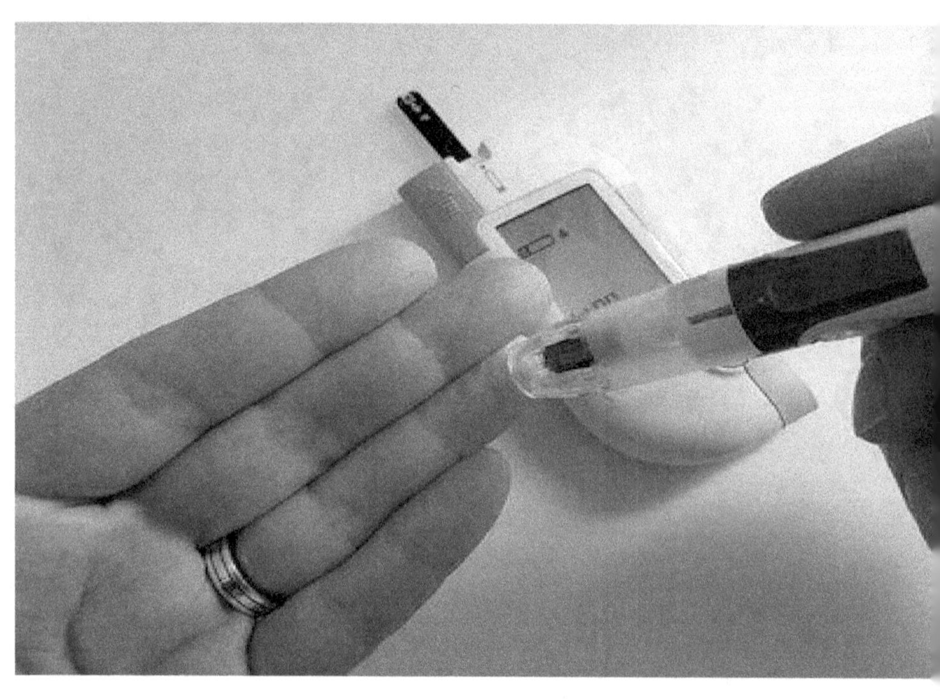

CHAPTER 6

A HEALTHY DIET

For overall health and wellbeing, eating a balanced diet that maintains optimal blood sugar levels is essential. To assist you in achieving that, below is a thorough meal plan for a blood sugar diet:

Recipe 1 for breakfast is one slice of whole-wheat bread.

almond butter, 1 tbsp

one boiled egg

1 little apple

1 cup of almond milk without sugar

Recipe 2

Oatmeal, half a cup

fresh berries in a cupful

a tablespoon of chopped nuts, such as walnuts or almonds

1 cup of almond milk without sugar

Recipe 3

A spinach, tomato, and feta cheese-topped two-egg omelet.

a single slice of whole-grain bread

1 little orange

1 cup of almond milk without sugar

Option 1 for a Snack: 1 tiny apple

almond butter, 1 tbsp

Alternative 2: A single little handful of young carrots

Hummus, 1 tablespoon

Choice 3 One hard-boiled egg

1 little orange

LUNCH Recipe 1

Chicken breast, grilled, weighing 3 ounces

1 cup of mixed greens salad including kale, spinach, and arugula

Cherry tomatoes, half a cup

1/4 cup of cucumber slices

1/4 cup of almond slices

Olive oil and vinegar dressing, 1 tbsp

Recipe 2

3 ounces of salmon, grilled

Roasted sweet potatoes, half a cup

1 cup of broccoli, steam-cooked

Olive oil and lemon juice dressing, 1 tbsp

Recipe 3

 One cup of lentil soup

Whole-grain bread, one slice

a half-cup of berries.

SNACK Recipe 1

1 little apple

1 tbsp almond butter Alternative

1 little bunch of baby carrots

1 hard-boiled egg Option 3 1 tablespoon of hummus

1 little orange

Recipe 1 for Dinner

a 3-ounce grilled steak and a half-cup of quinoa

1 cup of mixed greens salad including kale, spinach, and arugula

Cherry tomatoes, half a cup

1/4 cup of cucumber slices

Olive oil and vinegar dressing, 1 tbsp

Recipe 2

Chicken breast, grilled, weighing 3 ounces

1 tablespoon of an olive oil and lemon juice dressing, along with 1/2 cup of brown rice and 1 cup of steaming asparagus

Recipe 3

3 ounces of shrimp on the grill

quinoa, half a cup

Roasted Brussels sprouts in a cup with a sauce of olive oil and balsamic vinegar.

SNACK Recipe 2

1 little apple

almond butter, 1 tbsp

Recipe 3

1 little bunch of baby carrots

1 tbsp hummus Alternative 3

one boiled egg

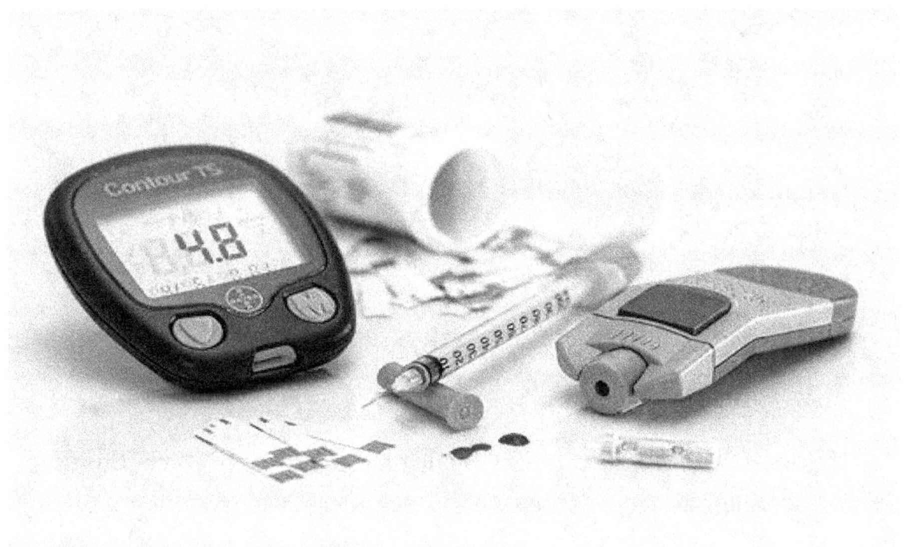

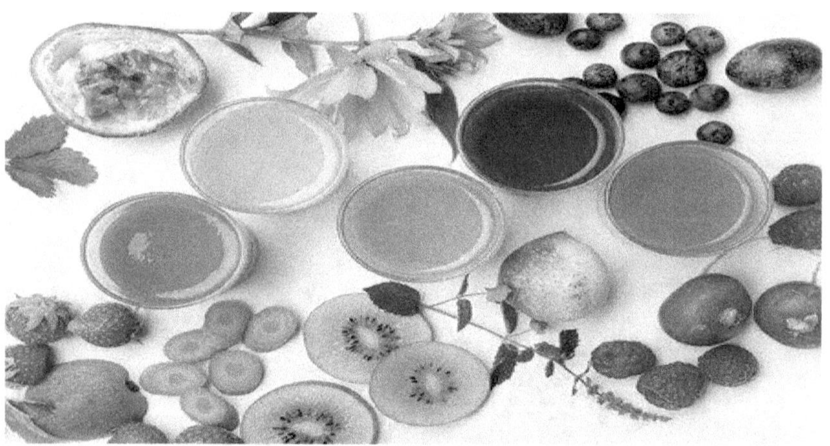

If you're just starting a blood sugar diet, it can be overwhelming to know where to start. Here's an 8-week meal plan to help get you on track:

WEEK 1

Day 1

Breakfast: Omelet with spinach, mushrooms, and feta cheese

Snack: Baby carrots and hummus

Lunch: Grilled chicken breast with mixed green salad

Snack: Apple with almond butter

Dinner: Grilled salmon with roasted asparagus

Day 2

Breakfast: Greek yogurt with berries and chopped nuts

Snack: Hard-boiled egg and orange

Lunch: Lentil soup with whole-grain bread

Snack: Baby carrots and hummus

Dinner: Grilled steak with mixed green salad

Day 3

Breakfast: Avocado toast with hard-boiled egg

Snack: Small handful of almonds

Lunch: Chicken and vegetable stir-fry with brown rice

Snack: Apple with almond butter

Dinner: Baked salmon with roasted sweet potatoes

Day 4

Breakfast: Smoothie with spinach, berries, and almond milk

Snack: Baby carrots and hummus

Lunch: Grilled chicken breast with mixed green salad

Snack: Hard-boiled egg and orange

Dinner: Grilled shrimp with roasted Brussels sprouts

Day 5

Breakfast: Oatmeal with almond milk, berries, and chopped nuts

Snack: Small handful of almonds

Lunch: Turkey and avocado wrap with mixed green salad

Snack: Apple with almond butter

Dinner: Grilled chicken breast with roasted vegetables

Day 6

Breakfast: Greek yogurt with berries and chopped nuts

Snack: Baby carrots and hummus

Lunch: Tuna salad with mixed green salad

Snack: Hard-boiled egg and orange

Dinner: Grilled steak with roasted asparagus

Day 7

Breakfast: Smoothie with spinach, berries, and almond milk

Snack: Small handful of almonds

Lunch: Grilled chicken breast with mixed green salad

Snack: Apple with almond butter

Dinner: Baked salmon with roasted vegetables

WEEK 2

Day 1

Breakfast: Avocado toast with hard-boiled egg

Snack: Baby carrots and hummus

Lunch: Turkey and avocado wrap with mixed green salad

Snack: Apple with almond butter

Dinner: Grilled salmon with roasted asparagus

Day 2

Breakfast: Greek yogurt with berries and chopped nuts

Snack: Small handful of almonds

Lunch: Chicken and vegetable stir-fry with brown rice

Snack: Hard-boiled egg and orange

Dinner: Grilled steak with mixed green salad

Day 3

Breakfast: Omelet with spinach, mushrooms, and feta cheese

Snack: Baby carrots and hummus

Lunch: Grilled chicken breast with mixed green salad

Snack: Apple with almond butter

Dinner: Baked salmon with roasted sweet potatoes

Day 4

Breakfast: Smoothie with spinach, berries, and almond milk

Snack: Small handful of almonds

Lunch: Lentil soup with whole-grain bread

Snack: Baby carrots and hummus

Dinner: Grilled shrimp with roasted Brussels sprouts

Day 5

Breakfast: Oatmeal with almond milk, berries, and chopped nuts

Snack: Baby carrots and hummus

Lunch: Tuna salad with mixed green salad

WEEK 3

Day 1

Breakfast: Greek yogurt with berries and chopped nuts

Snack: Hard-boiled egg and orange

Lunch: Turkey and avocado wrap with mixed green salad

Snack: Baby carrots and hummus

Dinner: Grilled salmon with roasted vegetables

Day 2

Breakfast: Omelet with spinach, mushrooms, and feta cheese

Snack: Small handful of almonds

Lunch: Grilled chicken breast with mixed green salad

Snack: Apple with almond butter

Dinner: Baked salmon with roasted sweet potatoes

Day 3

Breakfast: Smoothie with spinach, berries, and almond milk

Snack: Baby carrots and hummus

Lunch: Tuna salad with mixed green salad

Snack: Hard-boiled egg and orange

Dinner: Grilled steak with roasted asparagus

Day 4

Breakfast: Oatmeal with almond milk, berries, and chopped nuts

Snack: Small handful of almonds

Lunch: Chicken and vegetable stir-fry with brown rice

Snack: Baby carrots and hummus

Dinner: Grilled shrimp with mixed green salad

Day 5

Breakfast: Avocado toast with hard-boiled egg

Snack: Baby carrots and hummus

Lunch: Lentil soup with whole-grain bread

Snack: Apple with almond butter

Dinner: Grilled chicken breast with roasted vegetables

Day 6

Breakfast: Greek yogurt with berries and chopped nuts

Snack: Small handful of almonds

Lunch: Turkey and avocado wrap with mixed green salad

Snack: Hard-boiled egg and orange

Dinner: Baked salmon with roasted asparagus

Day 7

Breakfast: Smoothie with spinach, berries, and almond milk

Snack: Baby carrots and hummus

Lunch: Grilled chicken breast with mixed green salad

Snack: Apple with almond butter

Dinner: Grilled steak with roasted Brussels sprouts

WEEK 4

Day 1

Breakfast: Scrambled eggs with spinach and whole-grain toast

Snack: Greek yogurt with berries

Lunch: Tuna salad with mixed greens

Snack: Carrot sticks with hummus

Dinner: Grilled chicken with roasted vegetables

Day 2

Breakfast: Green smoothie with spinach, kale, berries, and almond milk

Snack: Small handful of almonds

Lunch: Lentil soup with whole-grain bread

Snack: Apple slices with almond butter

Dinner: Grilled salmon with roasted asparagus

Day 3

Breakfast: Greek yogurt with berries and chopped nuts

Snack: Hard-boiled egg and orange

Lunch: Grilled chicken salad with mixed greens and avocado

Snack: Carrot sticks with hummus

Dinner: Baked sweet potato with grilled shrimp and mixed vegetables

Day 4

Breakfast: Omelet with mushrooms, spinach, and feta cheese

Snack: Small handful of almonds

Lunch: Grilled chicken breast with mixed greens and balsamic vinaigrette

Snack: Apple slices with almond butter

Dinner: Grilled steak with roasted Brussels sprouts

Day 5

Breakfast: Avocado toast with hard-boiled egg

Snack: Greek yogurt with berries

Lunch: Tuna salad with mixed greens

Snack: Carrot sticks with hummus

Dinner: Baked salmon with roasted sweet potatoes and broccoli

Day 6

Breakfast: Green smoothie with spinach, kale, berries, and almond milk

Snack: Small handful of almonds

Lunch: Grilled chicken breast with mixed greens and avocado

Snack: Apple slices with almond butter

Dinner: Grilled shrimp with roasted vegetables

Day 7

Breakfast: Oatmeal with almond milk, berries, and chopped nuts

Snack: Greek yogurt with berries

Lunch: Chicken and vegetable stir-fry with brown rice

Snack: Carrot sticks with hummus

Dinner: Grilled chicken with roasted asparagus

WEEK 5

Day 1

Breakfast: Scrambled eggs with spinach and whole-grain toast

Snack: Greek yogurt with berries

Lunch: Chicken and vegetable stir-fry with brown rice

Snack: Carrot sticks with hummus

Dinner: Grilled salmon with roasted asparagus

Day 2

Breakfast: Green smoothie with spinach, kale, berries, and almond milk

Snack: Small handful of almonds

Lunch: Tuna salad with mixed greens

Snack: Apple slices with almond butter

Dinner: Grilled steak with roasted Brussels sprouts

Day 3

Breakfast: Greek yogurt with berries and chopped nuts

Snack: Hard-boiled egg and orange

Lunch: Grilled chicken breast with mixed greens and balsamic vinaigrette

Snack: Carrot sticks with hummus

Dinner: Baked sweet potato with grilled shrimp and mixed vegetables

Day 4

Breakfast: Omelet with mushrooms, spinach, and feta cheese

Snack: Small handful of almonds

Lunch: Lentil soup with whole-grain bread

Snack: Apple slices with almond butter

Dinner: Grilled chicken with roasted vegetables

Day 5

Breakfast: Avocado toast with hard-boiled egg

Snack: Greek yogurt with berries

Lunch: Chicken and vegetable stir-fry with brown rice

Snack: Carrot sticks with hummus

Dinner: Baked salmon with roasted sweet potatoes and broccoli

Day 6

Breakfast: Green smoothie with spinach, kale, berries, and almond milk

Snack: Small handful of almonds

Lunch: Grilled chicken breast with mixed greens and avocado

Snack: Apple slices with almond butter

Dinner: Grilled shrimp with roasted vegetables

Day 7

Breakfast: Oatmeal with almond milk, berries, and chopped nuts

Snack: Greek yogurt with berries

Lunch: Tuna salad with mixed greens

Snack: Carrot sticks with hummus

Dinner: Grilled steak with roasted asparagus

WEEK 6

Day 1

Breakfast: Scrambled eggs with spinach and whole-grain toast

Snack: Greek yogurt with berries

Lunch: Grilled chicken salad with mixed greens and avocado

Snack: Carrot sticks with hummus

Dinner: Grilled salmon with roasted asparagus

Day 2

Breakfast: Green smoothie with spinach, kale, berries, and almond milk

Snack: Small handful of almonds

Lunch: Tuna salad with mixed greens

Snack: Apple slices with almond butter

Dinner: Grilled steak with roasted Brussels sprouts

Day 3

Breakfast: Greek yogurt with berries and chopped nuts

Snack: Hard-boiled egg and orange

Lunch: Chicken and vegetable stir-fry with brown rice

Snack: Carrot sticks with hummus

Dinner: Baked sweet potato with grilled shrimp and mixed vegetables

Day 4

Breakfast: Omelet with mushrooms, spinach, and feta cheese

Snack: Small handful of almonds

Lunch: Lentil soup with whole-grain bread

Snack: Apple slices with almond butter

Dinner: Grilled chicken with roasted vegetables

Day 5

Breakfast: Avocado toast with hard-boiled egg

Snack: Greek yogurt with berries

Lunch: Grilled chicken salad with mixed greens and avocado

Snack: Carrot sticks with hummus

Dinner: Baked salmon with roasted sweet potatoes and broccoli

Day 6

Breakfast: Green smoothie with spinach, kale, berries, and almond milk

Snack: Small handful of almonds

Lunch: Grilled chicken breast with mixed greens and balsamic vinaigrette

Snack: Apple slices with almond butter

Dinner: Grilled shrimp with roasted vegetables

Day 7

Breakfast: Oatmeal with almond milk, berries, and chopped nuts

Snack: Greek yogurt with berries

Lunch: Tuna salad with mixed greens

Snack: Carrot sticks with hummus

Dinner: Grilled steak with roasted asparagus

Day 1

Breakfast: Scrambled eggs with spinach and whole-grain toast

Snack: Greek yogurt with berries

Lunch: Chicken and vegetable stir-fry with brown rice

Snack: Carrot sticks with hummus

Dinner: Grilled salmon with roasted asparagus

Day 2

Breakfast: Green smoothie with spinach, kale, berries, and almond milk

Snack: Small handful of almonds

Lunch: Tuna salad with mixed greens

Snack: Apple slices with almond butter

Dinner: Grilled steak with roasted Brussels sprouts

Day 3

Breakfast: Greek yogurt with berries and chopped nuts

Snack: Hard-boiled egg and orange

Lunch: Grilled chicken salad with mixed greens and avocado

Snack: Carrot sticks with hummus

Dinner: Baked sweet potato with grilled shrimp and mixed vegetables

Day 4

Breakfast: Omelet with mushrooms, spinach, and feta cheese

Snack: Small handful of almonds

Lunch: Lentil soup with whole-grain bread

Snack: Apple slices with almond butter

Dinner: Grilled chicken with roasted vegetables

Day 5

Breakfast: Avocado toast with hard-boiled egg

Snack: Greek yogurt with berries

Lunch: Chicken and vegetable stir-fry with brown rice

Snack: Carrot sticks with hummus

Dinner: Baked salmon with roasted sweet potatoes and broccoli

Day 6

Breakfast: Green smoothie with spinach, kale, berries, and almond milk

Snack: Small handful of almonds

Lunch: Grilled chicken breast with mixed greens and balsamic vinaigrette

Snack: Apple slices with almond butter

Dinner: Grilled shrimp with roasted vegetables

Day 7

Breakfast: Oatmeal with almond milk, berries, and chopped nuts

Snack: Greek yogurt with berries

Lunch: Tuna salad with mixed greens

Snack: Carrot sticks with hummus

Dinner: Grilled steak with roasted asparagus

WEEK 8

Day 1

Breakfast: Scrambled eggs with sautéed spinach and whole-grain toast

Snack: Small handful of almonds

Lunch: Grilled chicken and vegetable skewers with quinoa

Snack: Apple slices with almond butter

Dinner: Baked salmon with roasted Brussels sprouts and sweet potatoes

Day 2

Breakfast: Green smoothie with kale, spinach, berries, and unsweetened almond milk

Snack: Greek yogurt with berries

Lunch: Lentil soup with whole-grain bread

Snack: Carrot sticks with hummus

Dinner: Grilled shrimp with roasted vegetables

Day 3

Breakfast: Oatmeal with almond milk, berries, and chopped nuts

Snack: Hard-boiled egg and orange

Lunch: Grilled chicken salad with mixed greens, avocado, and quinoa

Snack: Apple slices with almond butter

Dinner: Baked sweet potato with grilled steak and mixed vegetables

Day 4

Breakfast: Veggie omelet with spinach, mushrooms, onions, and tomatoes

Snack: Greek yogurt with berries

Lunch: Tuna salad with mixed greens and quinoa

Snack: Carrot sticks with hummus

Dinner: Grilled chicken breast with roasted asparagus and cauliflower rice

Day 5

Breakfast: Green smoothie with kale, spinach, berries, and unsweetened almond milk

Snack: Small handful of almonds

Lunch: Chicken and vegetable stir-fry with brown rice

Snack: Apple slices with almond butter

Dinner: Grilled salmon with roasted vegetables

Day 6

Breakfast: Greek yogurt with berries and chopped nuts

Snack: Hard-boiled egg and orange

Lunch: Grilled chicken salad with mixed greens, avocado, and quinoa

Snack: Carrot sticks with hummus

Dinner: Grilled sirloin steak with roasted Brussels sprouts and mashed cauliflower

Day 7

Breakfast: Oatmeal with almond milk, berries, and chopped nuts

Snack: Greek yogurt with berries

Lunch: Tuna salad with mixed greens and quinoa

Snack: Apple slices with almond butter

Dinner: Baked sweet potato with grilled shrimp and mixed vegetables

NOTE

Remember to adjust portion sizes to meet your specific calorie and nutrient needs, and consult with your Doctor before starting any new diet or exercise program.

8-WEEK BLOOD SUGAR DIET MEAL PLAN FOR ADVANCED DIETERS

WEEK 1

Day 1

Breakfast: Vegetable omelet with spinach, mushrooms, onions, and tomatoes.

Snack: Greek yogurt with berries

Lunch: Grilled chicken salad with mixed greens, avocado, and quinoa

Snack: Carrot sticks with hummus

Dinner: Grilled salmon with roasted asparagus and cauliflower rice

Day 2

Breakfast: Green smoothie with kale, spinach, berries, and unsweetened almond milk

Snack: Small handful of almonds

Lunch: Chicken and vegetable stir-fry with brown rice

Snack: Apple slices with almond butter

Dinner: Baked sweet potato with grilled shrimp and mixed vegetables

Day 3

Breakfast: Greek yogurt with berries and chopped nuts

Snack: Hard-boiled egg and orange

Lunch: Tuna salad with mixed greens and quinoa

Snack: Carrot sticks with hummus

Dinner: Grilled chicken breast with mixed greens and balsamic vinaigrette

Day 4

Breakfast: Avocado toast with hard-boiled egg

Snack: Greek yogurt with berries

Lunch: Lentil soup with whole-grain bread

Snack: Apple slices with almond butter

Dinner: Grilled steak with roasted Brussels sprouts and quinoa

Day 5

Breakfast: Scrambled eggs with spinach and whole-grain toast

Snack: Greek yogurt with berries

Lunch: Grilled chicken salad with mixed greens, avocado, and quinoa

Snack: Carrot sticks with hummus

Dinner: Baked salmon with roasted sweet potatoes and broccoli

Day 6

Breakfast: Green smoothie with kale, spinach, berries, and unsweetened almond milk

Snack: Small handful of almonds

Lunch: Chicken and vegetable stir-fry with brown rice

Snack: Apple slices with almond butter

Dinner: Grilled shrimp with roasted vegetables

Day 7

Breakfast: Oatmeal with almond milk, berries, and chopped nuts

Snack: Greek yogurt with berries

Lunch: Tuna salad with mixed greens and quinoa

Snack: Carrot sticks with hummus

Dinner: Grilled steak with roasted asparagus and quinoa

WEEK 2

Day 1

Breakfast: Veggie scramble with spinach, mushrooms, onions, and tomatoes

Snack: Greek yogurt with berries

Lunch: Grilled chicken salad with mixed greens, avocado, and quinoa

Snack: Carrot sticks with hummus

Dinner: Grilled salmon with roasted asparagus and cauliflower rice

Day 2

Breakfast: Green smoothie with kale, spinach, berries, and unsweetened almond milk

Snack: Small handful of almonds

Lunch: Chicken and vegetable stir-fry with brown rice

Snack: Apple slices with almond butter

Dinner: Baked sweet potato with grilled shrimp and mixed vegetables

Day 3

Breakfast: Greek yogurt with berries and chopped nuts

Snack: Hard-boiled egg and orange

Lunch: Tuna salad with mixed greens and quinoa

Snack: Carrot sticks with hummus

Dinner: Grilled chicken breast with mixed greens and balsamic vinaigrette

Day 4

Breakfast: Avocado toast with hard-boiled egg

Snack: Greek yogurt with berries

Lunch: Lentil soup with whole-grain bread

Snack: Apple slices with almond butter

Dinner: Grilled steak with roasted Brussels sprouts and quinoa

Day 5

Breakfast: Green smoothie with kale, spinach, berries, and unsweetened almond milk

Snack: Small handful of almonds

Lunch: Chicken and vegetable stir-fry with brown rice

Snack: Apple slices with almond butter

Dinner: Baked sweet potato with grilled shrimp and mixed vegetables

Day 6

Breakfast: Green smoothie with kale, spinach, berries, and unsweetened almond milk

Snack: Small handful of almonds

Lunch: Grilled chicken and vegetable skewers with quinoa

Snack: Apple slices with almond butter

Dinner: Grilled salmon with roasted sweet potatoes and green beans

Day 7

Breakfast: Oatmeal with almond milk, berries, and chopped nuts

Snack: Greek yogurt with berries

Lunch: Tuna salad with mixed greens and quinoa

Snack: Carrot sticks with hummus

Dinner: Grilled sirloin steak with roasted asparagus and mashed cauliflower

Day 1

Breakfast: Scrambled eggs with spinach and whole-grain toast

Snack: Greek yogurt with berries

Lunch: Grilled chicken salad with mixed greens, avocado, and quinoa

Snack: Carrot sticks with hummus

Dinner: Baked salmon with roasted Brussels sprouts and sweet potatoes

Day 2

Breakfast: Green smoothie with kale, spinach, berries, and unsweetened almond milk

Snack: Small handful of almonds

Lunch: Chicken and vegetable stir-fry with brown rice

Snack: Apple slices with almond butter

Dinner: Grilled shrimp with roasted vegetables

Day 3

Breakfast: Greek yogurt with berries and chopped nuts

Snack: Hard-boiled egg and orange

Lunch: Tuna salad with mixed greens and quinoa

Snack: Carrot sticks with hummus

Dinner: Grilled chicken breast with mixed greens and balsamic vinaigrette

Day 4

Breakfast: Avocado toast with hard-boiled egg

Snack: Greek yogurt with berries

Lunch: Lentil soup with whole-grain bread

Snack: Apple slices with almond butter

Dinner: Grilled steak with roasted asparagus and quinoa

Day 5

Breakfast: Veggie omelet with spinach, mushrooms, onions, and tomatoes

Snack: Greek yogurt with berries

Lunch: Grilled chicken salad with mixed greens, avocado, and quinoa

Snack: Carrot sticks with hummus

Dinner: Baked sweet potato with grilled shrimp and mixed vegetables

Day 6

Breakfast: Green smoothie with kale, spinach, berries, and unsweetened almond milk

Snack: Small handful of almonds

Lunch: Chicken and vegetable skewers with quinoa

Snack: Apple slices with almond butter

Dinner: Grilled salmon with roasted asparagus and cauliflower rice

Day 7

Breakfast: Oatmeal with almond milk, berries, and chopped nuts

Snack: Greek yogurt with berries

Lunch: Tuna salad with mixed greens and quinoa

Snack: Carrot sticks with hummus

Dinner: Grilled sirloin steak with roasted Brussels sprouts and mashed cauliflower

Day 1

Breakfast: Veggie omelet with spinach, mushrooms, onions, and tomatoes

Snack: Small handful of almonds

Lunch: Grilled chicken and vegetable skewers with quinoa

Snack: Apple slices with almond butter

Dinner: Baked salmon with roasted Brussels sprouts and sweet potatoes

Day 2

 Breakfast: Green smoothie with kale, spinach, berries, and unsweetened almond milk

Snack: Greek yogurt with berries

Lunch: Lentil soup with whole-grain bread

Snack: Carrot sticks with hummus

Dinner: Grilled shrimp with roasted vegetables

Day 3

Breakfast: Oatmeal with almond milk, berries, and chopped nuts

Snack: Hard-boiled egg and orange

Lunch: Grilled chicken salad with mixed greens, avocado, and quinoa

Snack: Apple slices with almond butter

Dinner: Baked sweet potato with grilled steak and mixed vegetables

Day 4

Breakfast: Scrambled eggs with spinach and whole-grain toast

Snack: Greek yogurt with berries

Lunch: Tuna salad with mixed greens and quinoa

Snack: Carrot sticks with hummus

Dinner: Grilled chicken breast with roasted asparagus and cauliflower rice

Day 5

Breakfast: Green smoothie with kale, spinach, berries, and unsweetened almond milk

Snack: Small handful of almonds

Lunch: Chicken and vegetable stir-fry with brown rice

Snack: Apple slices with almond butter

Dinner: Grilled salmon with roasted vegetables

Day 6

Breakfast: Greek yogurt with berries and chopped nuts

Snack: Hard-boiled egg and orange

Lunch: Grilled chicken salad with mixed greens, avocado, and quinoa

Snack: Carrot sticks with hummus

Dinner: Grilled sirloin steak with roasted Brussels sprouts and mashed cauliflower

Day 7

Breakfast: Oatmeal with almond milk, berries, and chopped nuts

Snack: Greek yogurt with berries

Lunch: Tuna salad with mixed greens and quinoa

Snack: Apple slices with almond butter

Dinner: Baked sweet potato with grilled shrimp and mixed vegetables

WEEK 5

Day 1

Breakfast: Veggie omelet with spinach, mushrooms, onions, and tomatoes

Snack: Small handful of almonds

Lunch: Grilled chicken and vegetable skewers with quinoa

Snack: Apple slices with almond butter

Dinner: Baked salmon with roasted Brussels sprouts and sweet potatoes

Day 2

Breakfast: Green smoothie with kale, spinach, berries, and unsweetened almond milk

Snack: Greek yogurt with berries

Lunch: Lentil soup with whole-grain bread

Snack: Carrot sticks with hummus

Dinner: Grilled shrimp with roasted vegetables

Day 3

Breakfast: Oatmeal with almond milk, berries, and chopped nuts

Snack: Hard-boiled egg and orange

Lunch: Grilled chicken salad with mixed greens, avocado, and quinoa

Snack: Apple slices with almond butter

Dinner: Baked sweet potato with grilled steak and mixed vegetables

Day 4

Breakfast: Scrambled eggs with spinach and whole-grain toast

Snack: Greek yogurt with berries

Lunch: Tuna salad with mixed greens and quinoa

Snack: Carrot sticks with hummus

Dinner: Grilled chicken breast with roasted asparagus and cauliflower rice

Day 5

Breakfast: Green smoothie with kale, spinach, berries, and unsweetened almond milk

Snack: Small handful of almonds

Lunch: Chicken and vegetable stir-fry with brown rice

Snack: Apple slices with almond butter

Dinner: Grilled salmon with roasted vegetables

Day 6

Breakfast: Greek yogurt with berries and chopped nuts

Snack: Hard-boiled egg and orange

Lunch: Grilled chicken salad with mixed greens, avocado, and quinoa

Snack: Carrot sticks with hummus

Dinner: Grilled sirloin steak with roasted Brussels sprouts and mashed cauliflower

Day 7

Breakfast: Oatmeal with almond milk, berries, and chopped nuts

Snack: Greek yogurt with berries

Lunch: Tuna salad with mixed greens and quinoa

Snack: Apple slices with almond butter

Dinner: Baked sweet potato with grilled shrimp and mixed vegetables

WEEK 6

Day 1

Breakfast: Scrambled eggs with spinach and whole-grain toast

Snack: Small handful of almonds

Lunch: Grilled chicken and vegetable skewers with quinoa

Snack: Apple slices with almond butter

Dinner: Baked salmon with roasted Brussels sprouts and sweet potatoes

Day 2

Breakfast: Green smoothie with kale, spinach, berries, and unsweetened almond milk

Snack: Greek yogurt with berries

Lunch: Lentil soup with whole-grain bread

Snack: Carrot sticks with hummus

Dinner: Grilled shrimp with roasted vegetables

Day 3

Breakfast: Oatmeal with almond milk, berries, and chopped nuts

Snack: Hard-boiled egg and orange

Lunch: Grilled chicken salad with mixed greens, avocado, and quinoa

Snack: Apple slices with almond butter

Dinner: Baked sweet potato with grilled steak and mixed vegetables

Day 4

Breakfast: Veggie omelet with spinach, mushrooms, onions, and tomatoes

Snack: Greek yogurt with berries

Lunch: Tuna salad with mixed greens and quinoa

Snack: Carrot sticks with hummus

Dinner: Grilled chicken breast with roasted asparagus and cauliflower rice

Day 5

Breakfast: Green smoothie with kale, spinach, berries, and unsweetened almond milk

Snack: Small handful of almonds

Lunch: Chicken and vegetable stir-fry with brown rice

Snack: Apple slices with almond butter

Dinner: Grilled salmon with roasted vegetables

Day 6

Breakfast: Greek yogurt with berries and chopped nuts

Snack: Hard-boiled egg and orange

Lunch: Grilled chicken salad with mixed greens, avocado, and quinoa

Snack: Carrot sticks with hummus

Dinner: Grilled sirloin steak with roasted Brussels sprouts and mashed cauliflower

Day 7

Breakfast: Oatmeal with almond milk, berries, and chopped nuts

Snack: Greek yogurt with berries

Lunch: Tuna salad with mixed greens and quinoa

Snack: Apple slices with almond butter

Dinner: Baked sweet potato with grilled shrimp and mixed vegetables

Day 1

Breakfast: Scrambled eggs with spinach and whole-grain toast

Snack: Small handful of almonds

Lunch: Grilled chicken and vegetable skewers with quinoa

Snack: Apple slices with almond butter

Dinner: Baked salmon with roasted Brussels sprouts and sweet potatoes

Day 2

Breakfast: Green smoothie with kale, spinach, berries, and unsweetened almond milk

Snack: Greek yogurt with berries

Lunch: Lentil soup with whole-grain bread

Snack: Carrot sticks with hummus

Dinner: Grilled shrimp with roasted vegetables

Day 3

Breakfast: Oatmeal with almond milk, berries, and chopped nuts

Snack: Hard-boiled egg and orange

Lunch: Grilled chicken salad with mixed greens, avocado, and quinoa

Snack: Apple slices with almond butter

Dinner: Baked sweet potato with grilled steak and mixed vegetables

Day 4

Breakfast: Veggie omelet with spinach, mushrooms, onions, and tomatoes

Snack: Greek yogurt with berries

Lunch: Tuna salad with mixed greens and quinoa

Snack: Carrot sticks with hummus

Dinner: Grilled chicken breast with roasted asparagus and cauliflower rice

Day 5

Breakfast: Green smoothie with kale, spinach, berries, and unsweetened almond milk

Snack: Small handful of almonds

Lunch: Chicken and vegetable stir-fry with brown rice

Snack: Apple slices with almond butter

Dinner: Grilled salmon with roasted vegetables

Day 6

Breakfast: Greek yogurt with berries and chopped nuts

Snack: Hard-boiled egg and orange

Lunch: Grilled chicken salad with mixed greens, avocado, and quinoa

Snack: Carrot sticks with hummus

Dinner: Grilled sirloin steak with roasted Brussels sprouts and mashed cauliflower

Day 7

Breakfast: Oatmeal with almond milk, berries, and chopped nuts

Snack: Greek yogurt with berries

Lunch: Tuna salad with mixed greens and quinoa

Snack: Apple slices with almond butter

Dinner: Baked sweet potato with grilled shrimp and mixed vegetables

Day 1

Breakfast: Scrambled eggs with sautéed spinach and whole-grain toast

Snack: Small handful of almonds

Lunch: Grilled chicken and vegetable skewers with quinoa

Snack: Apple slices with almond butter

Dinner: Baked salmon with roasted Brussels sprouts and sweet potatoes

Day 2

Breakfast: Green smoothie with kale, spinach, berries, and unsweetened almond milk

Snack: Greek yogurt with berries

Lunch: Lentil soup with whole-grain bread

Snack: Carrot sticks with hummus

Dinner: Grilled shrimp with roasted vegetables

Day 3

Breakfast: Oatmeal with almond milk, berries, and chopped nuts

Snack: Hard-boiled egg and orange

Lunch: Grilled chicken salad with mixed greens, avocado, and quinoa

Snack: Apple slices with almond butter

Dinner: Baked sweet potato with grilled steak and mixed vegetables

Day 4

Breakfast: Veggie omelet with spinach, mushrooms, onions, and tomatoes

Snack: Greek yogurt with berries

Lunch: Tuna salad with mixed greens and quinoa

Snack: Carrot sticks with hummus

Dinner: Grilled chicken breast with roasted asparagus and cauliflower rice

Day 5

Breakfast: Green smoothie with kale, spinach, berries, and unsweetened almond milk

Snack: Small handful of almonds

Lunch: Chicken and vegetable stir-fry with brown rice

Snack: Apple slices with almond butter

Dinner: Grilled salmon with roasted vegetables

Day 6

Breakfast: Greek yogurt with berries and chopped nuts

Snack: Hard-boiled egg and orange

Lunch: Grilled chicken salad with mixed greens, avocado, and quinoa

Snack: Carrot sticks with hummus

Dinner: Grilled sirloin steak with roasted Brussels sprouts and mashed cauliflower

Day 7

Breakfast: Oatmeal with almond milk, berries, and chopped nuts

Snack: Greek yogurt with berries

Lunch: Tuna salad with mixed greens and quinoa

Snack: Apple slices with almond butter

Dinner: Baked sweet potato with grilled shrimp and mixed vegetables

Remember to adjust portion sizes to meet your specific calorie and nutrient needs, and consult with a healthcare professional before starting any new diet or exercise program.

BONUS

EASY EXERCISES THAT DIABETIC PATIENTS CAN DO TO CONTROL AND MANAGE BLOOD SUGAR

Walking

Walking may be done practically anywhere and is a terrific low-impact exercise. Start out with easy strolls and gradually build up to longer and more vigorous walks.

Swimming

Another low-impact activity that is easy on the joints is swimming. It is a fantastic approach to increase endurance and cardiovascular health.

Yoga

Yoga is a gentle kind of exercise that helps increase strength, flexibility, and balance. Additionally, it helps to lower stress and enhance general wellbeing.

Cycling

Cycling is a fantastic aerobic workout that can be done both inside and outside. Both blood sugar levels and heart health are improved.

Resistance Exercise

Building muscle mass and enhancing insulin sensitivity can be accomplished by resistance exercise, such as weightlifting or the use of resistance bands.

Dancing

A fun method to stay active and enhance cardiovascular health is to dance. Additionally, it helps with coordination and balance.

Tai chi

Tai chi is a gentle exercise that incorporates deep breathing and leisurely motions. It can aid in enhancing flexibility, balance, and stress reduction.

Pilates

Pilates is an exercise method that emphasizes strengthening the muscles in the core. It can aid in enhancing flexibility, balance, and stress reduction.

Chair workouts

Low-impact workouts called "chair exercises" can be performed while seated. Seniors and anyone with mobility challenges will love these.

Stretching

A fantastic technique to increase flexibility and lower the chance of injury is by stretching. It doesn't need special equipment and can be done anywhere.

Exercising Aerobically

Jogging, running, or brisk walking are examples of aerobic exercises that can help with weight loss, blood sugar control, and cardiovascular health.

Interval training

Resistance training and aerobic activities are combined during circuit training. It is a fantastic technique to work out the entire body quickly.

Hiking

Hiking is a wonderful activity for getting outside and exercising. Blood sugar levels can be brought down, and cardiovascular health can be improved.

Aquatic exercise

Exercise that has a low impact and is easy on the joints is water aerobics. Stress reduction and cardiovascular health can both be helped by it.

Calisthenics

Bodyweight exercises like calisthenics can be performed anyplace. Push-ups, squats, and lunges are a few of the activities that are included in it; they can aid to increase strength and enhance insulin sensitivity.

Golfing

Walking and pushing or carrying a golf bag are both low-impact exercises that are involved in golf. Stress reduction and cardiovascular health can both be helped by it.

Rowing

On a rowing machine or in a boat, rowing is a low-impact activity. It aids in enhancing endurance and cardiovascular health.

Gardening

It's a terrific way to enjoy the outdoors and get some exercise via gardening. It entails exercises that can increase strength and flexibility, such as weeding, planting, and digging.

A stair ascent

A wonderful technique to improve leg strength and get some aerobic activity is to climb stairs.

9 7 9 8 3 9 2 5 5 8 6 9 8